The
Midp♥int
Plan

The
Midp•int
Plan

Gabby Logan

PIATKUS

PIATKUS

First published in Great Britain in 2024 by Piatkus

3 5 7 9 10 8 6 4 2

A CIP catalogue record for this book
is available from the British Library.

ISBN 978-034943-939-6

Printed and bound in Great Britain by
Clays Ltd, Elcograf S.p.A.

Papers used by Piatkus are from well-managed forests
and other responsible sources.

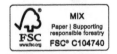

Neither the publisher nor the author is engaged in rendering
professional advice or services to the individual reader. The ideas,
procedures, and suggestions contained in this book are not intended as
a substitute for consulting with your doctor. All matters regarding
your wellbeing require medical supervision.

Piatkus
An imprint of
Little, Brown Book Group
Carmelite House
50 Victoria Embankment
London EC4Y 0DZ

An Hachette UK Company
www.hachette.co.uk

CONTENTS

PART THREE:
WHAT IS HAPPENING IN OUR LIVES?

INTRODUCTION

God grant me the serenity
to accept the things I cannot change,
the courage to change the things I can,
and the wisdom to know the difference.

REINHOLD NIEBUHR

We can thank the Canadian psychoanalyst Elliott Jaques for coming up with the concept of a 'midlife crisis'. He was studying the working lives of creative geniuses, when he noticed a pattern emerging in their attitudes at a certain age and he said that the midlife crisis was 'a time when we come face to face with our limitations, our restricted possibilities and our mortality'. Shamefully, I admit that my podcast *The Midpoint* – perhaps my answer to avoiding a personal midlife crisis – was the product of a moment of vanity and a little despair.

It was the late summer of 2019. I walked past a mirror, glanced over, and noticed that I had developed some strange lines around my cheeks. Thinking it must be the light, I moved. It wasn't the light. Now I could see that where once I'd had cute dimples there was a visible reminder that the juiciness of youth had all but gone: the dimples had morphed into lines. Dimples disappear when the smile is released. At least they used to. These lines stayed put. As I stared at this new (old) face in the mirror, I realised it was no longer reflecting me, the person inside. I was still full of vim and vigour, ideas and projects and, above all, full of life; I was still thirty inside. I'd turned forty without any signs of anxiety at all: age is just a number, right?

But these lines got me thinking about my age (forty-six at the time) and about what else was about to change in my body. What I hoped for more than a line-free face was a body that could carry out the wishes of my mind, one that wasn't about to start breaking down. In that discombobulating moment I heard a loud clock ticking in my head, heralding the news that it was highly likely (even with a family trait of living to be one hundred years old) that I was over or around midway through my life. I was at The Midpoint. Time was running out, or at least running away. *You are probably closer to death than birth*, I told myself. Then a mild panic set in. I hadn't written that sitcom set on a breakfast TV show which I'd been mulling over for years. I hadn't run a marathon. I hadn't been to Sweden. I hadn't written a book. All I could think about was what I hadn't achieved.

Then the flip side . . . I knew more stuff than my twenty-year-old self and was more confident in listening to my gut for answers than ever before. Dare I say it, I felt wiser and more grounded than at any time in my life. On good days I would even say I was content. In the weeks after this reverse eureka moment I started observing other midlife people more closely. I became somewhat obsessed. I noticed the ones whose dreary clothes and lacklustre bearing suggested they were resigned to their fate; and then there were those who were skipping through the day with energy and gusto, still relevant in their cultural and sartorial choices, still at the top table of life's decision makers, displaying bountiful positive energy. I knew which camp I wanted to be in, but I also wondered what happens to people to send them in one direction at The Midpoint crossroads of life. Why did some who were once full of hope and vitality fall into comfy and easy, while a life a bit more fulfilled and challenging was still an option at the crossroads? I'm well aware that statement is loaded with my bias. Who is to say that comfy and easy is wrong?

All of life is a choice. Sure, we are dealt a certain genetic hand, but we can hack into our destiny with positive life decisions, and taking the more proactive route at The Midpoint crossroads was the choice for me. I'd always said, when asked by beauty journalists, that I wasn't going to be someone who succumbed to facelifts, wasting thousands of pounds trying to hold back Father Time. I love facials and I have always paid attention to my skin, but the 'no facelift for me' attitude was delivered somewhat cockily, when I still had ample amounts of collagen and bounce-back ability in my skin. Bounce-back ability is when you have a big night out and the morning after, when you've consumed a couple of cups of coffee and had a quick run round the block, you are as a good as new. That doesn't happen after forty.

I am not currently contemplating a facelift to chase youth – each to their own, however – but I realised that a lot of what I had previously read or focused on was about the aesthetics of ageing, not what it really meant to be a healthier, more productive, creative and happy older person. I was very determinedly marching down this road of midlife when I started to notice things happening or not happening as they should. The physical: my skin was starting to look dry in a strange crêpey way; my hair was a little bit more unruly; my periods were becoming much less frequent; I wasn't getting the same results from exercise, muscle seemed harder to maintain; the same food had a different effect on me, and also alcohol as previously mentioned. The mental: my previously photographic brain was often failing me – occasionally on live TV; I was becoming shorter tempered with my family; I was anxious; I woke up more at night and my normally positive demeanour was sliding into something more cynical.

Fortuitously I had already started recording my podcast *The Midpoint*, which I have previously described as the most self-serving podcast currently in the charts, the premise being: woman who works in the media hits midlife and then sets about recording a podcast to explore what well-known and interesting people are doing about it. The idea had come to me in 2019 (around the time of the aforementioned mirror moment) but it took a global pandemic for me to get my arse into gear and start recording the first series. I set about texting interesting famous people in my address book who were in the correct age bracket (thirty-eight to sixty, according to the Economic and Social Research Council), especially those who had done something inspiring in midlife, and then I'd interview them. Each episode would also feature an expert who would deliver their wisdom on a range of midlife topics.

John Bishop was the very first guest. At the age of forty and with three young sons, he had given up a steady well-paid job as a salesman for a pharmaceutical company to become a stand-up comedian. When I interviewed him, he was fifty-six and globally successful in that second career. Next up was Denise Lewis, the Olympic gold-medal-winning heptathlete, who at forty-seven had given birth to her fourth child. I realised quite quickly that I knew a lot of interesting midlifers and hoped that their stories might appeal to the midlife community. Around eight episodes in I interviewed Mariella Frostrup, the broadcaster and journalist who is ten years ahead of me on the midlife journey, and who had just co-written a book about the menopause. Until that day I had naively thought the symptoms of ageing I described above were just that, me getting older. The fact that I had never had a hot flush or night sweats meant to my mind that I wasn't menopausal. Well, it turned out, as I listened to Mariella, that my 'symptoms' weren't all about ageing – they clearly related to perimenopause. I didn't even know that was a thing! I was woefully under-educated about the perimenopause and about the symptoms my midlife body was experiencing.

Something was happening in wider society regarding this midlife phase and in the first 2020 lockdown a generation of people who had been lucky enough to forge careers often in the media and the arts (i.e. they had a voice and an audience) were of an age that they saw some physical and mental changes occurring and they began to talk. Careers were paused because of Covid and time was abundant, there was a stillness to life which meant we began to notice, to pay more attention to ourselves. It was a perfect storm. For many folk like me, we initially blamed the more subtle mental symptoms that appeared on the lockdown. Surely that's why I was anxious and increasingly bad tempered? No, not entirely, as it transpired; I probably needed my diminishing hormones topping up, but more on that later.

The conversations got louder and more public and it felt as though the menopause taboo was slowly being lifted. But this was not just an issue for women. As I dug deeper into the menopause and midlife generally, I could see that this was a period of life which needed a rebrand. Men also dealt with diminishing hormones, though not at the same rate as women, and have other health concerns and mental challenges. According to suicide stats for 2021 from the Office for National Statistics, three-quarters of all suicide is male and the biggest age bracket is forty-five to forty-nine. Yet middle-aged men and women have been portrayed in comedically tragic tropes for as long as I can remember. The bloke who buys a Ferrari and leaves his wife for a younger woman; the woman whose menopausal symptoms leave her angry, hot (in temperature) and often single, having once been the wife of Ferrari man. Of course, real life has presented us with examples of both and everything in-between (my own parents split up at the age of fifty-two so I had a fine example of how midlife can present challenges in a long relationship), but reality is much more nuanced.

Whether we navigate the choppy waters of our relationships or jump ship, the middle years of our lives should be some of the best. We have often brought up and sent our kids into the world by this point and time becomes ours to play with once more; our financial situation should be at its healthiest (if we have careers, our peak earning power will usually be in our fifties); and if we look after ourselves we have the possibility to do all we did in our twenties with very few of the insecurities.

But we can't 'positive mindset' our way out of the facts; there is science to contend with, our bodies are changing, and the risks of certain diseases and illnesses are increasing. How we navigate the next few decades could determine whether we spend our seventies and beyond sedentary and on medication or thriving and climbing hills with people we love and in relationships that are still nurturing. Even if you are picking this book up today as a late forty-something who has taken their eye off nutrition and the exercise routine has fallen by the wayside, it is not too late. Do not give up on yourself as being too old to change; if there is one thing I would love you to come away with it is that message.

As Greg Whyte, the Olympic pentathlete (who has gone on to be a world-record-breaking swimmer and coach to many celebrities on Comic and Sport Relief challenges) said on a *Midpoint* episode, 'Start lifting weights today, it is never ever too late to start.' Lifting weights is known to be one of the most important protectors against osteoporosis and heart disease and its importance will come up a few times over the course of this book.

I want every reader of this book to feel supported, and encouraged to grow, plan and thrive. As I recorded more and more *Midpoint* episodes, I realised that there was a mine of information and experiences that I needed to share with a wider audience and I wanted to write the book *I* needed when I was heading into this midlife period: a book I could keep by my bed, pick up, flick to the chapter that pertained to my feelings that day or the issue that seemed to be consuming me that week and find some comfort, motivation and maybe a shared experience. I feel good about life and in myself as I approach fifty-one years old, and when I have rubbish days, I feel I can deal with them so much better than I did in my twenties and thirties, and this is largely down to the habits and practices I have adopted and nurtured, many taken from the hundreds of guests I've talked to since I started *The Midpoint*. As a result, there's a smorgasbord of wisdom and experiences which will work for some and not for others. Many of my guests have adopted things which don't suit me – for example, the comedian Lee Mack's best efforts to convince me to become vegan didn't work – but they might work for you. By the way, I did commit to eating a lot more vegetarian food after I spoke to him, so he has changed my habits.

We can't turn back time, but we can work towards our best possible future. I hope this book will bring you a clearly mapped-out blueprint to navigating the biggest topics that hit us at midlife. It is divided into three key areas: what is happening in our heads, our bodies and our lives. I wanted to bring together in one place the best of the hours and hours of conversations I have been having on *The Midpoint* podcast on topics important to you, me and everyone in and around the midlife. I've been lucky enough to gather invaluable learnings from the brilliant experts I have interviewed on things that worry, confuse or sometimes torment us at this time in our life. If you have been feeling unsure about how you are going to cope with an empty nest, for example, I want you to know that there are some great years ahead but you might need to make a plan; if you have no motivation to exercise, I want you to finish this book believing that it must become one of the most important habits you adopt – and I know when you hear how it will future proof your body you will want to get moving as soon as you can.

Interwoven throughout, of course, will be my own stories, explaining how I am dealing with all the changes I, Kenny and my family are experiencing as we make our way from young to older. There are other voices on these pages, too – in the following chapters are funny, moving and heart-warming stories from a wonderful array of actors, musicians, sports legends, politicians, business leaders and more, on what happened – or is happening – to them in those decades of great change, their forties, fifties and sixties. With honesty and humour, they've shared anecdotes you'll find reassuring and helpful.

I want you to take away useful advice, anecdotes and action plans and see The Midpoint as a time to thrive not just to survive. I've written it as something you can dip in and out of when issues or questions arise; to be kept on your bedside table, on the shelf in the kitchen or in the loo. Now, to begin on the next stage – possibly the best stage – of your future. Good luck to that, and let's get reading.

PART ONE

What is happening in our minds?

1 MENTAL PERFORMANCE

Do not dwell in the past, do not dream of the future,
concentrate the mind on the present moment.

BUDDHA

For me the journey into midlife and beyond has to be holistic –
mind, body and soul – the most important of which, in my
opinion, is the mind. I've got no interest in having a line-free face
if I can't recall a name, or tight abs if I can't read more than two
pages of a book without being distracted. This is why I've given just
as much attention to keeping my brain performing well, investing
time and making changes to help my memory, mindset and motivation stay strong, as I have given to my face in the mirror or my
abs in the gym. And this is why I've made all things related to the
mind the opening section of this book.

For those of us who work, our professional lives will provide at
least some mental stimulus. Even if you have stopped working you
will get your mental stimuli in other ways – family, hobbies, sport,
volunteering. However it is that we are spending our time and
using our brain, we may have noticed the way we handle certain
mental challenges has changed in the last few months or years.
Does remembering a name seem harder? Is it taking you longer
to recall the title of a song you love when it's playing on the radio?
Are you feeling a little distracted in conversations with friends?

Now, I love my work and I intend to do it for as long as I can, so the idea that it might be my mental performance, or lack of it, which might end my career was not something I ever wanted to contemplate. I'd always assumed, working in the shallow world of telly, that it would be my wrinkles. Would my mind hold me back from being able to continue to be professional, alert and motivated at work? It was one of the scariest things I began to consider as I entered The Midpoint; but I had to, because my mind was starting to change.

One of the first signs that I was reaching that midpoint stage of life – although I didn't know it at the time – was an unfamiliar brain fog. Around my mid- to late-forties I was increasingly struggling to recall facts as quickly as I used to. As I nearly always had a phone to hand, I would often search for the answer on it rather than let my brain work it out. At first, I didn't really notice that my brain wasn't doing it. Professionally it was noticeable that I couldn't research and write as quickly as I had done in the past, and then a few times when I was on live telly, I failed to recall the correct word or name and bluffed my way through the situation. It was an unfamiliar and unpleasant feeling; at one point I thought my brain might be full. I put this down to tiredness at first, but after a couple of alcohol-free weeks with optimum nutrition and eight hours' sleep a night, I was still feeling like a sub-standard version of myself.

The menopause is dealt with in much more detail in Chapter 9, but it was only by working out that my brain fog was possibly a symptom of perimenopause that I was able to do something about it. One of those things for me was talking to a doctor and eventually getting on hormone replacement therapy. Briefly, as it matters in relation to mental performance and this chapter, oestrogen is the hormone commonly recognised to help memory, learning and cognitive function, through the protection of nerve endings in the hippocampus. When it starts to diminish in women during perimenopause, these areas can be affected. A lowering of progesterone can also cause memory issues. Testosterone (which is produced by the ovaries in women and the testes in men) also contributes to mental sharpness. Most men do not experience a dramatic drop-off in testosterone in the way women do, so I also boosted my testosterone levels. I think it's important to say that not all women can or want to take HRT so there is a whole range of things we can do to help menopause symptoms which we can address later.

Once we understand what is going on with our brains at this point of our lives, everything becomes easier to manage. And it isn't just hormones. It may take longer to learn and recall information for a plethora of reasons, e.g., certain parts of the brain shrink as we get older; blood flow to it may decrease; neurons may be less effective; the effects of decades of stress, smoking and drinking may start to be felt more acutely. We need to use every tool we have to keep our memory and motivation working for us. I have made a few very conscious lifestyle decisions to protect my mental performance.

CHANGES THAT WORKED FOR ME AND MY MENTAL PERFORMANCE

I try to avoid reaching for the phone when I am struggling with an answer to a question or a name. Even if it takes me a few minutes, I need to let my brain have a go and work harder. This only works with people who know me well in social situations; I am fairly sure after about two seconds on telly someone would shout the word down my earpiece to avoid the viewer turning off.

I started playing an instrument. Well, I was bought a recorder for my fiftieth birthday, which is a good starting place if you are low in musical confidence – and it has reacquainted me with 'Frère Jacques'. I also got my old piano books out and tinkled away, but there didn't seem to be as much enthusiasm in the house for this.

Decreasing screen time is so impactful; we spend years telling our teenagers to put their phones down and actually we could do with practising what we preach. Like everyone, I fall down a social media rabbit hole occasionally and end up mindlessly scrolling utter nonsense. Thirty minutes could disappear after I initially picked up my phone to text someone ... which I then forgot to do. It is not just the waste of time whereby I could be learning or reading, or talking to my kids; I am sure it is not helping my attention span. Now, from time to time I delete those addictive apps and then a week or so later, if I have to post for work or a charity, I go back on and realise that life was probably better and more productive in those seven days disconnected. It's worth monitoring your behaviour and being honest with your usage just to see if it makes a difference.

I tried to learn to play chess, which didn't go very well. And then I joined a book club, which went better. I have always enjoyed reading but I recognised that I wasn't reading books that were outside my comfort zone. Also, I had a habit of reading about six chapters and then starting another book so I rarely finished anything. I became aware of the sphere of influence I was exposing myself to so I started listening to podcasts and reading articles and books which challenged my views. I was noticing that social media algorithms push people into silos, so they only receive information that's aligned to their already entrenched views. If I am listening to something which challenges my views I really have to think about the opposing argument, which is what we are taught most of the way through school and university and yet that habit seems to slip off as we age. The most interesting older people I speak to are ready for a robust debate and won't take it personally if they can't convert me to their way of thinking.

Back to protecting my mental performance, here's a really simple one: if I am paying someone online and sending money to a new bank account, I try to remember the seven-digit number in one go. The tiny wins are sometimes the most impactful. I suppose

I was subconsciously at first trying to do things that were going to help the performance of my brain by stretching it beyond what was easy. As a sports person I understood that to gain strength we lift heavier than before or to gain endurance we run further, so I pushed my brain like a muscle.

The Midpointer View

Lorraine Kelly, the ebullient TV broadcaster, has hosted her morning show for over two decades and at the age of sixty-four shows no signs of slowing down. I was really excited to have Lorraine on the podcast because she has been such a champion of women's health issues on her eponymous show and she was very open about her own midlife and menopause experiences. She told me how she appreciates that to stay on top in broadcasting, she has to keep her mind sharp. 'No one is indispensable. I never take my career for granted . . . every day is a school day, and I am still so curious, I love the research I have to do for my guests, the books and the films I need to consume. In order to be interesting, you have to be interested.' Her work keeps her sociable, too – another plus when it comes to keeping your mind happy in midlife and beyond. 'It's a joy I can talk to people properly. Keep being curious, keep being interested. Your brain will respond in such a positive way. And I think that is a youthfulness, isn't it? Which you can have whatever age you are, your attitude.'

FOOD FOR THOUGHT

We'll discuss diet and nutrition more specifically in Chapter 5, but I found that small incremental changes are likely to be the wins which are vital in forming better habits. So, a few years ago, when those perimenopausal symptoms started to kick in, I looked at my diet and supplementation, and started to take magnesium, which helps with energy levels, because if tiredness is a problem, then memory and cognitive function will inevitably suffer.

I also upped my intake of oily fish. Omega 3 is important throughout life for brain function but I didn't think it would do any harm to eat more fish and especially if that was at the expense of meat.

Here's a great tip when you embark on a new eating habit, such as bringing in three portions of oily fish into your weekly diet. According to James Clear in his book *Atomic Habits*, a change in habit is much more likely to stick if it is identity-based as opposed to outcome-based. For example, if you are eating the fish with the mindset, 'I am hoping to improve my mental performance,' it might not be as successful in becoming a regular habit as if you said to yourself, 'I eat oily fish because I am someone who has sharp mental performance.'

When Patrick Holford, one of the most highly regarded nutritionists in the world, published a book titled *Optimum Nutrition for the Mind*, he looked at how diet affects all aspects of the brain. It's a really powerful read, with the science to back up what my mum always said to me as a kid: 'Eat those sardines up and you'll do better at school.'

THE GOOD NEWS

Mental performance, for me anyway, is so closely aligned to self-esteem that I was happier and more positive in all areas of life when I felt I was able to keep doing the things I wanted to, and within a few weeks of taking the hormones, I noticed a difference: I felt more like me in the TV studio and then more engaged with the world beyond work. And the little tricks I've taught myself are helping me to focus and stay sharp, too. And of course, a midpoint brain isn't all bad. Perhaps contrary to its reputation as a slower version of the youthful brain, the middle-aged mind not only has the ability to maintain functionality but it can acquire new abilities, too – which is fantastic news.

'There is an enduring potential for plasticity, reorganization and preservation of capacities,' according to the cognitive neuroscientist Patricia A. Reuter-Lorenz, of the University of Michigan, in her paper with Joseph A. Mikels, *The Aging Mind and Brain: Implications of Enduring Plasticity for Behavioral and Cultural Change*. Even better than that, researchers from the Seattle Longitudinal Study, which tracked the cognitive abilities of adults over fifty years, showed middle-aged adults performed better on four out of six cognitive tests than those same individuals did as young adults. The same group of people *improved* with age.

Studies on pilots and air-traffic controllers – people you'd hope are razor sharp – show positive results in overall performance even if speed and memory capacity declined in older pilots. In 2007 a study published in *Neurology* (Volume 68, No. 9) tested pilots from forty to sixty-nine years of age on flight simulators, and while the older pilots took longer to learn to use the simulator, they eventually did a better job than younger colleagues in avoiding collisions, which would seem to be the ultimate win for a pilot, I'm sure you'd agree.

The middle-aged brain is becoming increasingly interesting to scientists, which is good news for those of us in the thick of it. By understanding why some middle-aged brains start to shut down while others present like those of a thirty-year-old, researchers are hoping that more people will have good mental performance in old age. There are undoubtedly some genetic variants that are risk factors for memory as we age, but in the Seattle study it was found that people who continue to show cognitive improvement in midlife also tend to be more physically, cognitively and socially active than those who don't fare as well. I read that as we have to keep moving, thinking and partying.

MATURE STUDENTS

Alexis Willett is the co-author of a book called *How Much Brain Do We Really Need?* and she knows just why health is worth prioritising, and why we all need to school ourselves. 'Ultimately the brain is at the core of everything we are and do. It's very easy to forget about it because it's inside us and we tend to focus on what our skin or hair looks like, and how our body is feeling. But we really need to work our brain in the way we work our bodies and keep mentally healthy as well as physically healthy. As we age, our brains just aren't as efficient in the way that our bodies just aren't as efficient. Things are a little more sluggish and it takes a bit more time for messages to pass through the brain between the neurons, to make connections and to lay down memories. Everything just takes a bit more effort ... '

So, what should we do? Go back to class?

'The brain is very plastic, very adaptable, but slightly less so as you get a bit older,' says Alexis. 'Challenging ourselves is critical for making new connections. Studies have shown that learning for enjoyment, for fun, might offset damage and help us to retain our cognitive function, and build a cognitive reserve – a pool of brain power that can help limit the damage as we age. The longer you stay in education, or just push yourself mentally, the higher your cognitive reserve will hopefully be when you're older. It's not as easy as just doing a crossword every day – that's great, keep going – but as clinical neuropsychologist Dr Fergus Gracey says, it would be equivalent to going to the gym and doing weights on one bicep every day and then going out to a football field and expecting to be great at football. It doesn't work like that. So, if you're regularly doing crosswords, you're getting great at crosswords, and you're just getting one little bit of your brain honed. What you need to do is challenge yourself to do something different and something that involves lots of parts of the brain.'

Alexis' big tip

- Read more books. 'You could think about joining a book club. You'll be exposed to a much wider range of books that challenge what you normally read. You'd be expected to think about a book and then convey your thoughts, using reasoning to talk about it. You're using social skills. It's about trying to find activities that really work right across the brain. Those that help you stay mentally curious and open. So, expose yourself to new experiences. Try new challenges. Don't limit yourself.'

MOVE YOUR MIND

Exercising the body can exercise the brain – as yoga teacher and wellness coach Mia Togo understands. 'I studied psychology at UCLA and did a deep dive into therapy and self-reflection. I was a professional dancer back in the eighties. I struggled with some of the typical things, body image and worthiness. And so, I made a pact with myself at a young age to do whatever I needed to do to deconstruct.' This promise she made to herself has helped her face the mental challenges of reaching The Midpoint. Lessons she's learnt include:

- Stay connected. 'Connecting to your body and really listening to what it wants is key to keeping motivated and mentally active.' Go for a walk in the forest, dance to your favourite eighties classic, or wake up and do stretches. Moving the body helps motivate the mind.
- Everyone can have a bad day – but don't give up. 'I think the typical thing for many people is feeling like they get momentum, and then something derails them, and they feel like they're back at ground zero.' Don't let it. Push forward. Start again. There are no limits to how many times you can begin an exercise regime or healthy eating plan. Keep going until it becomes routine. Tomorrow is a new day.
- We all need positive self-talk. So many people have the desire to move forward and 'go towards the things that light them up (but get) stuck in this rut of negative thinking,' Mia warns. Stop it. Shut down those conversations and tell yourself you are still smart, you can finish a project, you can remember that fact, etc.
- Practise gratitude. When Mia started to feel grateful for her body – moving and stretching it with consistent yoga practices, even if just for five minutes a day – her brain lit up as well. 'It's helped support me – not just my physical body [but] my mind, my heart, because in yoga it's all connected.' Putting in the effort to stay fit and supple reaps mental rewards, too.
- 'You need to make space for yourself. And sometimes there's this shame or this guilt of like I'm being selfish

or self-centred. And this is the time, more than ever, to really take your sovereignty back.'

When it comes to your mind in midlife, we can *all* do more than we think, with a few tweaks, changes, kind words to ourselves – and maybe a trip to the doctor, whether we're male or female, if we suspect our hormones are messing with our heads.

MIDPOINT ACTION POINTS

- Have more fun and games to keep your brain active, or take up a new hobby. Try to do crosswords, word searches or Sudoku puzzles. Regular crossworders show a slower decline in cognitive ability than the rest of the population on average. Jigsaws are great cognitive sharpeners because they encourage total focus and work both sides of the brain. Take up chess – the ultimate problem-solving game.
- Give yourself time to find the answer to something before you reach for the mobile phone and google it. Take a beat, it's in there. The warm glow of satisfaction when you realise you do know the answer is worth it.
- Lifestyle changes are key. Take a look at your diet and try to add a few portions of oily fish. Also if you are deficient in vitamin B complex this can lead to brain fog, so you might need a supplement. If in doubt always ask your doctor for advice. And move more. We too often associate exercise with the body and how we look, but scientists know now it is just as important for the mind and how we feel (more on this in Chapter 4) – and if you can do it outside, all the better for reducing cortisol,

boosting endorphins and blowing away any cobwebs that may have accumulated in your brain.

- Talk to yourself the way you would talk to a friend – with kindness, understanding and encouragement. Yes, your mind and mental performance may be changing but it doesn't mean you're washed-up or useless, you just have some adapting to do.

2 MIDLIFE CRISES

This is not the end. This is not even the beginning of the end. But it is, perhaps, the end of the beginning.

SIR WINSTON CHURCHILL

The traditional 'sitcom' version of a midlife crisis used to be represented by a man (or, if the writers are very modern, a woman) who buys something too fast to drive, loses weight and gains hair and eventually runs off from his wife and family to be with a younger, more voluptuous and nubile woman. To which another male character sitting in a bar on hearing the story of said bloke will quip, 'And what's the crisis?'

Unsurprisingly the term seems to have attracted a negative association, because nobody likes the idea of being the bloke in the sitcom or of admitting to a crisis. But it may please you to learn that the term midlife crisis has its roots in something much more solid and academic than a throwaway joke to make people aged between forty and sixty feel bad about themselves. As I shared in the introduction, it was first written about in 1965 in a research paper by the psychoanalyst and social scientist Elliott Jaques, called *Death and The Midlife Crisis*. When he first read out his work to a group of peers and academics – Jaques had described a midlife crisis as 'where we come face to face with our limitations, our restricted possibilities and our mortality' – they didn't think he was on to anything. What do you think as a midlife person reading this book? His analysis might sound a tiny bit pretentious . . . but pretty spot on, right?

In the fifties, though, the psychoanalysts of the world weren't ready for it and Jaques took another seven years to publish his ideas, by which point he had captured the zeitgeist. People were feeling it, and his ideas were making it into the mainstream – even if mainly as gags in family comedies. Without wanting to get all Sociology GCSE here, it seems because of their privilege in having careers and money, the early idea of a midlife crisis seemed only to apply to middle-class white men, who'd hit something of a career plateau and had lots of new leisure time available to sit around wondering what was the point in it all. The working class didn't have the luxury of time to worry about a midlife crisis and often died younger anyway. Women were too busy with marriage, menopause and kids to notice if they were having one, apparently. But do not fear, women and the working class were not excluded for long, because medical and technological advancements and social reform meant more rights and opportunities, so before long it was acknowledged that they too were succumbing to the effects of a midlife crisis.

Throughout the 1990s there was a school of thought that we were in the grip of a self-fulfilling prophecy when it came to midlife. If we told ourselves that this would be a time of upheaval and worry and questioning then we would probably experience all of that, but the choice was ours. If we could reframe this period of our lives and tell ourselves midlife would be a time for opportunity, and focus on the many joys of getting older, then we could experience a much more positive period of our lives. Choose to have a crisis or choose joy – was it really that simple?

Now, I am all for positivity and reframing, but I feel the reality is probably somewhere in the middle of Elliott Jaques' doom-and-gloom paper and the 1990s take on the midlife crisis, which was to pull yourself up by your bootstraps and plaster a smile on your face.

There is no doubt that the physical changes we experience have an effect in terms of the way we feel about ourselves mentally – we can no longer push ourselves to do the things we once took for granted, and that's depressing. Plus, we're reaching the age when friends start to get ill and die, and that forces us to acknowledge that time is indeed running out; we are closer to death than birth and we still have some pretty big decisions to make and questions to answer ... Is this the relationship I want to stay in for ever? Do I want to keep trudging up this career path for the next twenty years? Are these my friends for life? Am I happy? All pretty big questions.

My parents spilt up on the day of my thirtieth birthday party when they were fifty-two and fifty-three years old. There is a heavy back story to their eventual divorce, including the death of my brother, but I did see plenty of evidence that at least one of them was refusing to settle for something that was unhappy and unfulfilling. I don't think it was a crisis, but I *do* think there is something about the energy needed to uproot and rebuild and we probably know deep down that we might not have that same energy in fifteen years' time, so best get on with it. We also know that looking for a new partner might be easier with a couple of decades on our side.

The crisis might not be directly related to your relationship; it could be professional – a desire to escape the rat race, perhaps, or to retrain and do something totally different. How we frame this period of life will definitely have an impact on how successfully we navigate it: crisis or opportunity? Only you can decide.

The Midpointer View

Let's start on a positive note about what happens after the midlife crisis from Kerry Godliman, the stand-up comedian and actress beloved for her roles in Ricky

Gervais' *After Life* and *Derek*. 'I'm assured by friends in their fifties that life gets better in your fifties – once you get over that hump. I think the forties are very turbulent, especially the late forties with the menopause and being on the precipice of being that big Five O. And then once you've got that behind you, I'm led to believe it gets really good and that you suddenly have all your energy back and certain things are understood.'

Going back to Jaques' 'we have restricted possibilities' analysis, he has a point. When you are twenty-five years old, there are fewer restrictions to contemplate, especially if you are single, mortgage-free and childless. Taking a job on the other side of the world is as easy as packing a bag and booking a flight. Ending an unhappy relationship can be tough in the moment but if you both appreciate it is for the long-term best, and you're living alone or renting to-gether – and have no kids – you can avoid a massive drama. Scroll on twenty-five years with kids, bills, baggage, and you can easily make excuses for being less nimble and staying put in a situation which doesn't make you happy.

My husband Kenny and I loved buying and doing up houses in our thirties; we moved seven times in a decade. In the year of my fortieth birthday, we bought our biggest project to date and we haven't moved since. At times I think this is because we are settled, enjoying the home and loving our neighbours, but there are moments when doubts slip in. Are we staying put because I have got a little bit comfy and the idea of uprooting is exhausting? Am I coming face to face with my limitations? In spite of my public protestations of feeling no different to thirty-eight-year-old me, I think she might have moved us all on to a new project by now. It's a dilemma when I ask myself if I am more mature and accepting now, or if I am settling for what I have got.

The Midpointer View

Radio DJ and TV presenter Jo Whiley admitted to me, 'It's a challenging time of your life, I will say that. I do, I definitely think that it's very complicated because you have so many things that you are having to deal with, whether it's your children growing up or your parents getting older, your advancing years, the changes when you look in the mirror. All these things mess with your head. But there's also a power in the age that you are and the experience you've got and the knowledge that you have in your head. It's a time to take stock of what is important to you and to just keep on keeping on.' I grew up admiring Jo as a broadcaster; she's only a few years older than me but when I was a young upstart on local radio, she was a star of BBC Radio 1 and I have always admired the passion she exudes for music when she broadcasts. She's eternally cool and relevant in a genre which, obsessed with youth, could so easily have spat her out. To hear her talk about her midlife doubts and frustrations made me admire her even more.

ASKING THE QUESTIONS ... AND BEING OKAY WITH THE ANSWERS

I have been having some kind of 'questioning' episode – if not a full-blown crisis – for the last few years. This is how I am handling this new stage of my midlife:

- Taking it day by day, or decade by decade. I feel since turning fifty I have started to look at my life in little chunks of time. By the time we are fifty-five years old, Kenny and I will have kids who are twenty-three, which seems a reasonable age to assume they can't complain if we wanted to up sticks and move to a different part of the country, on the basis they might well be working in Australia or Canada should they choose. At the moment my eighteen-year-old son loves the part of the world we live in so much he has threatened to never come home if we leave it. Which has both positive and negative ramifications. Looking at my life in these time chunks has stopped my brain from worrying too much about the distant future, and totally unravelling.

- Allowing room in my life to ask questions. Over the last few years, especially during the pandemic, I could be found typing things like 'is my law degree still relevant' into my Google search engine. Did I really want to become a barrister? Probably not, but I was asking myself lots of questions. How can my job help anyone? What use am I? This was not the first time I had realised my profession as a 'sports broadcaster' had limited benefits for society. One Christmas back in the early 2000s when Kenny and I were still footloose and fancy-free, we volunteered for a Crisis at Christmas shelter in the East End of London. The form-filling is quite thorough and there were a lot of questions included to ascertain what use you'd be to the homeless people making use of the facility. Doctors, nurses, counsellors and therapists, hairdressers, physios, podiatrists, massage therapists and lawyers were all very useful to those who'd be staying for a few days; a sports broadcaster and her rugby-playing husband less so. We were assigned 'general use', which meant lots of chatting and making cups of tea, which was apparently useful too.

- Once the pandemic panic had subsided, I was able to

look at the pros and cons of my current life with a clear head. I have enormous respect for people who gear change in midlife and retrain or make a big move; very few regret the changes. But what I realised after all of my questioning, and when I eventually went back to work as the restrictions eased, was that I loved my job and that I was hitting my peak years. This wasn't the time to quit and change but a time to embrace all the experiences I had enjoyed and seize the opportunity to say 'yes' to projects I had avoided before because of the children and their school-bound lives.

- Not throwing the baby out with the bathwater, but making tweaks to enhance my current midlife set-up. I didn't become a barrister obviously, but I did push myself in other ways and tried new things. I started my podcast and wrote a book, things I had been procrastinating about for years. I said yes to a TV show that made me fall in love with cold water therapy and eventually conquer a fear of heights by jumping off a 400ft bridge (with a safety harness, of course, or I probably wouldn't be writing this).

- Using my questioning as a way to make the most of every minute. I guess my crisis didn't mean I had to sell my house or leave my husband to find the answers, it was about realising what there was left to do, not regretting the years that had gone by.

- Owning my shit. When you've come through the other side of questioning all your decisions, you really know who you are and what is important, and it makes you stronger. I have more clarity about what I stand for, and I know not to be silenced or apologetic. My Midpoint self-questioning has given me that.

The Midpointer View

Sports presenter Andrew Cotter is one of my favourite colleagues, and on *The Midpoint* we had a really interesting conversation about midlife crises, and about the decisions and changes life springs at us around this point. I told him about an article that stated how important the age of forty-seven is: that if you hadn't achieved your goals by forty-seven you never would, because that's your disposition cemented, and you're going to stay in that zone for the rest of your life. I asked him if he believed that, and felt that forty-seven was a pivotal age for him (he was born in 1973) – and for all of us. 'This time of life is when we say it's the crossroads, it's now or never … it is absolutely now or never,' he told me. 'And you get this sort of existential angst about it all and say, Is this what I do? Is this what I am and I'm going to be forever more? And what is my purpose and what am I? And so, you think, Right, I'll do this and it might work. The worst thing to do would be to look back and say, I wish I'd tried. I wish I'd taken a little bit of a leap. And if it didn't work, it didn't work. But at least I had a little glimpse at what was out there, what was possible.'

And he confessed the thought of ageing may be giving him a little midlife crisis of his own. 'People say, "Oh, I'm looking forward to growing old disgracefully. It's going to be fantastic." Well, it's not, I just don't see that at all because a lot of it is a physical thing in that I have loved sporting activity, and I still run but my hips hurt a bit now, something that didn't happen ten years ago. Everything starts falling apart. Your teeth start falling out and your hair goes. If you say you're looking forward to that ... come on now. Really?' Did I mention he's also famously comically dour.

DIVERT A CRISIS, MAKE A CHANGE

Frances Edmonds, author of *Repotting Your Life: Reframe Your Thinking. Reset Your Purpose. Rejuvenate Yourself Time and Again*, is a longevity and well-being fellow at Stanford University's Distinguished Careers Institute, and knows a lot about living through and getting over a midlife crisis – or a time of intense reflection and questioning – both professionally and personally.

'I was mindlessly watching this gardening show, and the commentator picked up this pot and it had this withered old, sad little languishing plant in it. And he pulled it out and the roots were going round and round in a tight little ball, and he said, "This plant is pot bound. It's run out of nutrients in its environment. It's no longer flourishing, and unless I repot this plant, it's going to wither and die." And I thought, Oh my God, I am pot-bound! And it does tend to happen at a certain age, doesn't it? Because you've gone through some various life landmarks, whether it is having a family or getting married, or getting divorced, then with that feeling of getting older, physically or mentally.'

HOW DO YOU REPOT YOURSELF?

'Some things you can't change, like if somebody dies or you have an incurable illness,' says Frances. 'I call those black hole problems. And the only thing you can do about those is change the way you respond to them or the way you're thinking about them, but other things you can change.' We talk more about how to handle and adjust to black hole problems in a later chapter on loss, but for now, when you can take control, Frances has great tips on finding a new way to flourish in midlife:

- First of all, when you've identified that you are pot bound, you have to name it – you have to say, Why is it I'm not feeling right? Often, it's not easy to articulate what it is. So, you have to do some work. Am I not living my authentic life, or is this relationship not working? Do I have a bad pattern? I'm eating too much, or I'm drinking too much; I'm not working enough or I'm working too much.
- When you've named that pattern, you can start to tame it. When you understand what it is, at that point, you can start reframing it. Do I really want to sit in bed all day watching Netflix? Do I want to sit in this useless relationship or this bad job? Or do I want to do something about it? So that is the first part of the process.
- Then you have to uproot from your old life and move into another situation. And that's tough. That's when you have a look at the skillset you've got and your transferrable talents. I think particularly with a lot of women they just think, Oh, I'm just a mother and a homemaker. But when you look at the skillset you need to keep all that afloat, they could be running a FTSE 100 company!
- Face the frightening stuff. There's a fear to change, and not just to a place, it can be a situation you're in, like someone being in a rubbish relationship or a job that doesn't suit them. It's like a baby's nappy. It's warm and comfortable, but it's toxic. But nothing worth doing is easy. When you want to do deep stuff on yourself, it's

going to cost you. When you uproot, you have to make a plan. Do an inventory of the skills you've got, then find the gaps, then fill them. You're starting at the bottom of the ladder with an open, beginner's mindset.

- Ask for guidance – you're never too old to need help. In all humility, ask people to give you ideas, feedback and help. Frances went through this process and lived her own repotting journey. 'I'd had various transitions in my life, but as I hit deep middle age, nothing was working. As the old Zen saying goes, when the student is ready, the master will appear . . . and some friends of mine said, "We are off to Stanford to be part of a cohort of twenty-five fellows from all over the world, with a programme based on wellness and purpose and community, want to join us and see what happens?" Not everybody can uproot themselves, leave Notting Hill, go off to Stanford and do that. Take those boring little steps to change – *get rid of my car, rent out my house, find a US bank, find an American accountant* – but when you have a big goal that motivates you, it keeps you going.'

- Don't forget to look back and congratulate yourself. Repotting at this stage of your life is hard. 'Eventually, you'll look back and think, How did I manage all of that? How did I get here? And those are confidence-building measures for the next time you want to repot and do something else. Because you know, the thing is, it never ends. If you have a growth mindset, it will keep you living longer, fitter, healthier – mentally, physically, spiritually and emotionally. It revives you like the plant that's been repotted.'

THREE MUST-HAVES TO NAVIGATE A MIDLIFE CRISIS

1. Humility. 'The humility not to think I'm the big deal,' advises Frances. 'I will start at the bottom again and I will learn. That's humility.'
2. Humanity. 'An openness and a curiosity about people, and an understanding that every single person can teach you something. Inclusivity is the policy, and diversity will then be the outcome.'
3. Humour. 'Because you can't change the facts of your life, but you can change the way you look at them.'

AGE IS ONLY A NUMBER

I had an interesting chat with the infamous truth teller Piers Morgan about how it felt to *not* be young any more. He spent so many years of his career being described as the young gun, the whippersnapper of the newsroom. 'Well, it's been interesting for me and a strange trajectory where the thing that I used to dislike is now the thing I crave most. When I was a newspaper editor, I was always considered incredibly young. I became editor of the *News of The World* at twenty-eight, then the editor of the *Daily Mirror* at thirty, so I was always being categorised as Boy Wonder, Wonder Kid, all that kind of thing, which actually got quite annoying after a while. I was like, "Hang on, I'm here. I'm married. It's not just because I'm young." So being called young all the time became something I didn't particularly like. And then as I got older, I began to realise how much I missed being called young.'

How was he handling middle age and did he have any advice to share on ageing and averting a midlife crisis, seeing as he's a decade ahead of me? His answer seems to be . . . denial! 'You get to, like, forty-five, fifty, and nobody ever again calls you Boy Wonder or Wonder Kid. In fact, quite the opposite. I have a theory that when you look in the mirror, you never see anybody over thirty. It doesn't matter how old you are, I've just noticed since the age of thirty, I always think I look thirty. And it's only when you meet other people your age, my village mates, for example, and I look at them and go, "God, you look old." And they laugh and go, "What about you? You're an old git." Suddenly you just don't see yourself in the way other people do. And I think as you age more from forty to fifty, and I assume as you get even older, you continue to see somebody a lot younger when you look at yourself in the mirror – and you're not.' So, if living in denial when you look at your reflection gets you though the day, so be it.

MIDPOINT ACTION POINTS

- These years can be tough and confusing. Everyone in your age bracket is probably feeling it. Don't become a victim, or look to blame others for your feelings of inertia or regret. It's all about you. Yes, other people can be a pain or a drain, but it's all about how you react to them. The only thing you have control over in this life is your response to it.
- Take stock of what you want to change so you can repot yourself, be it professionally or personally. Keep a to-do list, write ideas down in a journal, read books that will set you up for success (ahem, like this one – so you're on the right track), make a mood board, and tell people about your aims and goals. All these things will help hold you to account in a positive way, rather than letting you slip back into despair.

- Don't make rash decision in a flash or boredom or because you're just a bit fed up. Don't chase cool or follow a trend, think carefully about what you need. Know your options and think forward to all possible outcomes. Sometimes it's difficult to turn back the clock, so before you leave your partner, get a neck tattoo or buy the sports car you can't afford, consider it carefully.
- Don't be too self-critical if and when things don't go to plan. That's life in all its messy, beautiful, exhausting ways. Instead of being self-critical, become self-aware — learn from your mistakes, then move on.

3 MENTAL HEALTH

Although the world is full of suffering, it is also full of the overcoming of it.

HELEN KELLER

Most of us will experience periods of our lives where we feel overwhelmed and unable to cope with seemingly simple tasks. If we are lucky, that feeling may last a day or two; for others the anxiety deepens and the mental health dip lasts longer, sometimes resulting in depression and other mental illnesses. Thankfully we live in a world where the conversation about mental well-being is fairly widespread, and the taboo is lifting, although we are not yet perfect in quickly getting help for people who have serious issues, and more work needs to be done in all aspects of our society. Do seek help and book an appointment with your GP if you have issues you need to discuss.

For me, mental health has always been closely aligned to my physical well-being, and I feel we have to remind ourselves to be aware of that strong connection. In the same way we wouldn't expect our body to be able to go and run a marathon tomorrow without training, why do we expect our mental health to be constantly in perfect balance without attending to it?

Our mental health can be challenged at any age, but it wasn't until I started delving into this midpoint time of life that I learnt some pertinent facts. According to NHS statistics, for example, it is women in midlife who are the group of people most likely to be prescribed anti-depressants in the UK; and a study published in *Psychological Medicine* in 2021 revealed that British adults experienced their highest levels of psychological distress in their forties and fifties, with symptoms including anxiety and depression. In the study by University College London's Centre for Longitudinal Studies, at midlife 23 per cent of women and 17 per cent of men had mental ill health, higher than at other times in their adulthood. Reasons suggested for this include many topics we'll talk about in the book: empty nest syndrome, divorce, caring for children and older relatives, as well as job-related stress.

I found all of this particularly concerning (and sad!). It felt so unfair that when we've worked so hard for decades at this point – we've brought up families, and juggled jobs and careers for so long – we deserve a break. People shouldn't be feeling so wretched *just* at a time when they should finally be able to care for themselves a bit more, realise the wisdom they have accrued through all of life's travails and then enjoy the fruits of their labour.

We will discuss the menopause later in the book, a major player in mental health issues at midlife, but in this chapter, we will focus on the anxiety and low mood that can affect everyone at this point, when everything can feel a bit too much – caring for the generations above and below, accepting more responsibility at work, and perhaps dealing with new health issues that creep in as you hit your forties.

I had always been a positive, upbeat person, who understood the effect of good diet and exercise on my mood, and yet none of my usual tricks were working with the same impact any more. A big run didn't seem to deliver enough endorphins to see me through the day. I wasn't just unenthusiastic; I was also a bit snappy and angry. Now, being angry for the *right* reasons can be a middle-aged woman's super power, but being furious because the dishwasher hasn't been emptied or because someone forgot to put the washing on is a recipe to make the rest of your household want to avoid you for the night at best – and divorce you at worst.

MIDLIFE MELTDOWN

One day I was so cross about some low-level Sunday-morning apathy for household duties I told my gang I was considering moving out into my own flat in a nearby town. I delivered the speech as if I had researched it already, when it was actually a knee-jerk reaction to too many plates and mugs being left in a teenager's bedroom. Instead of feeling better and achieving any kind of balance, I had the kids close to tears and my poor husband wondering where his positive, upbeat wife had gone. I didn't feel better for this outburst. In my previous life as a regularly menstruating woman, I would say I was capable of getting fired up and a bit irrational every couple of months, so there was an obvious link to my menstrual cycle. But now it was anyone's guess how I would respond to an innocuous domestic disappointment. I didn't want to be an unnecessarily shouty woman for the rest of my days.

The doctor I saw was a specialist in women's health – the first time I'd visited anyone like this since I was pregnant – and she immediately recommended that I rebalance my hormones, which I decided to do with great joy ... and joy is what returned very quickly to my life. Of course, everyone is different. Some women may still need antidepressants in the fifty to fifty-nine-year-old bracket, but a great many might not. The ratio of men to women taking them would certainly indicate that there is further research needed and better help from and for the medical profession.

MEN NEED MATES

There is of course a positive in women even heading off to the GP in the first place and that's the willingness to discuss what is going on with their mental health. Women appear to find it easier to open up to someone and ask for help before things get too bad. Men sadly take much more drastic action, and a few take their own life. Men, it seems, still need to be encouraged to talk. My own husband Kenny recognised this after we experienced the death of a dad from school. One week this lovely man was on the sidelines shouting encouragement to the boys playing rugby, the next he was dead. You hear the statistics and the stories about how quickly mental health can deteriorate, but this was a brutal reminder to us. It transpired that this man's decline had happened over a matter of weeks not years.

I noticed Kenny become very proactive in keeping various groups of friends together, booking in social and sporting events and picking up the phone and calling when he felt one of the group was a bit quiet. He also started a regular Monday-morning phone call with his best man who lived a few hundred miles away, which seemed mutually beneficial. In one of his social groups there were three divorces out of five men in a matter of years, and the times they spent talking and supporting each other really impressed me. Men need mates; if you are married to one or care about one, I would say that is one thing you can actively encourage. Kenny often walks with another group of men and again I know they have much more personal chats on the walks – perhaps it's easier than sitting face to face in a pub or bar.

We discuss Kenny's prostate cancer diagnosis later in the book but I think his openness about that and what happened next has led many men (some of whom he has never met) to contact him with their own concerns or to seek reassurance if they are about to have their prostate removed. A problem shared is often a problem halved.

FILLING AN EMPTY TEAPOT

It can be hard even to think about putting yourself first at this point in your life, when you're running around after your kids or your elderly parents – but you must! Looking after your own mental health is not selfish. You can't pour tea from an empty teapot. In the midlife, more than ever, you need to give yourself the time and space – and permission – to do things just for you, your sanity and your stability. I've included here a few things I've started to do that have really boosted my mental health – and the science backs up the benefits, I feel.

TAKE THE PLUNGE

I have always known the power of exercise and diet when it comes to my mental well-being, but over the last few years I have added in to that mix 'cold water', whether that's swimming with my girlfriends in a lake on a Sunday morning, jumping into a freezing ice bath or just having a cold shower. I don't really need to know why it works; I just know it does. But for those who like to understand the science, many studies have shown that cold exposure can activate the sympathetic nervous system and increase the blood level of beta-endorphins as well as noradrenaline, which is a hormone vital in dealing with stress and anxiety. Getting into a freezing cold lake on a cold December morning is awful at first, the cold never fails to shock, but the mood-boosting effects afterwards are more than enough reward and the fact I have done something uncomfortable and pushed myself seems to work for me in a way which is difficult to quantify mentally. Bear in mind that cold-water exposure comes with risks so familiarise yourself with these before you give it a try.

The Midpointer View

Midpoint guest Davinia Taylor, former Hollyoaks actress and now a bestselling author, has written extensively on diet and its relationship with our moods and she is also a fan of a bit of cold water. 'I would recommend cold showers. I'm not very good with cold, so I generally have a hot, hot bath beforehand to the point where you can feel your pulse in your head. Twenty minutes sat in a hot bath, get out, have a cold shower for fifteen to twenty seconds and watch your hormones rebalance. You go into fight or flight mode. And then the parasympathetic nervous system calms you down when you realise you're not dying and you'll have some really nice, happy hormonal feelings. And that's the easiest way to start balancing your hormones and listening to your body. I also flip a coin. So, if it's heads, I go in the shower, that way I keep my body guessing; it's not a routine.'

It's clear that wild swimming, cold-water bathing, daring yourself to take a freezing plunge – even if it's just a thirty-second cold shower every morning – boosts mental health in many very real ways:

- Cold water gives a quick release of endorphins, serotonin and cortisol, all perfect for boosting a low mood.
- Swimming is gentle on ageing joints, gives hearts and lungs a good workout, and water resistance helps to build muscle and lowers blood pressure.
- The weightlessness of water has a calming effect on the mind, and the breathing patterns adopted during a swim

regulate brain waves, which in turn reduces anxiety, although I would say the water would need to be a little bit warmer to get a calming effect while you are actually in it.

- Sea water is brimming with minerals – magnesium, chloride, calcium and more – which help skin conditions like psoriasis and eczema. Sea swimming also reduces inflammation in the nose and throat.

- If you can't face getting into cold water, go out for a walk and breathe it in. Blue is the colour of peace and calm, bringing those benefits to an overworked brain; the rhythmic flows of the tide soothe the soul; while the sounds of waves chill out our nervous system.

GET OUTSIDE INTO NATURE

Perhaps the easiest, quickest mental health boost you can give yourself is to get outside. When I go for a long walk in the woods or countryside with my dogs, I stop as my dogs are sniffing something and find myself admiring a tree that has stood for a few hundred years, or I notice the dappled sunlight glinting through the tree-tops onto some crocuses that have made it through the ground, and I really take it in and express my gratitude for all these beautiful natural wonders. We all know the health benefits of being in nature, but it's taken me until my midlife to fully realise the power of the spiritual connection. Reconnecting with nature is free, easy and abundant, even for busy midlifers who can't quite set up a regular schedule at the gym.

Author of *Forest Therapy: Seasonal Ways to Embrace Nature for a Happier You*, Sarah Ivens spent twelve months, in her forties, studying and living the benefits of reconnecting with the great outdoors, discovering why and how a connection with the natural world helps create a sense of deeper meaning in our everyday midpoint life. Here's what she found out (through research and by adapting her daily habits) during the year:

- Research reported in *Environmental Science and Technology* found a link between decreased anxiety and bad moods with increased time in nature, and another study published in *Public Library of Science* proved immersing yourself in the wonders of the outdoors boosted creativity.
- A group of international psychologists published a paper in the *Journal of Environmental Psychology* explaining that being in touch with Mother Nature helps us to connect with our fellow humans too, making us kinder and more generous to those around us.
- Getting out into natural light boosts our vitamin D and serotonin levels and regulates our circadian rhythm (or body's internal clock) meaning we sleep better, which in turn eases feelings of sadness and sluggishness that can stop us from feeling positive about what lies ahead.
- It's a fact that taking in the sights, sounds and smells of a forest, a lake, a mountain or the sea fills us with feelings of awe, gratitude and wonder – reminding us in the most beautiful and fragrant ways that we are part of something much bigger than our work inbox or arguments over the laundry.

THINK YOURSELF TO A HEALTHIER MINDSET

The power of language cannot be underestimated. If we tell ourselves that our brains are slower, then they probably will be. We need to reframe our thinking and look at the opportunities we have to improve our mental health and cognitive ability.

Noor Hibbert is a life coach and bestselling author of *Just*

F*cking Do It: Stop Playing Small. Transform Your Life and believes we can learn to manifest a positive mindset, which is the ultimate tool for a good midlife and avoiding a midlife crisis. Our brains still have the power to change, but if you tell yourself, I am never going to be able to do this, you are creating that future. In other words: speak kindly to yourself . . . manifest improvements. Don't give up on your goals. 'There is always a *why* to a mindset and until you train your mind to think a certain way and answer the *why* you will not get the results.

'The first point I try to make to *everybody* is that everything we do in our life is a product of the thoughts we have. So, everything that we see in our physical world, all of the external that we see out here, are all the result of what's going on in the mind. And that's something that I had to learn, in my early twenties when I was really struggling with my mental health and not feeling like I had any control over it. Starting to understand that the thoughts that we have in here, that's the beginning of everything out there.'

The Midpointer View

Rugby legend Gareth Thomas shares some great advice about keeping your mental health on track, especially when it comes to handling criticism and flattery. 'I always remember a great friend of mine, a guy I played rugby with, called Glen Webbe and he was the first black man to play for Wales and I remember him saying to me after my second game, "You'll play for Wales one day. The only advice I will give you is when you start reading the good press; read the bad press," and it's stuck with me. It's a balance. I used to read negative reports and it would motivate me not to be that bad next week or motivate me to make sure that whoever wrote that couldn't write

the same next week because I was that much better.'
Very few of us reading this will be playing international
sport, but Gareth's advice applies to all of us: we are our
own worst critics but nothing is ever as bad or as good
as it seems.

Noor's tips for midlife self-improvement
and mental nourishment

- Look at your life. Ask yourself, What am I not
  happy with? What's happening up here? What is that
  thought? Are they negative? Do they lack confidence or
  motivation? 'Reverse engineer it back to the thoughts
  that we actually have about that thing to start off with,'
  advises Noor. 'That's usually a great place to start to
  realise, Okay, there's a bit of a path here, from that
  negative thought to where I am right now. So let me try
  and flip that.' Expect more of yourself. Nobody else is
  going to jump inside your head and tell you that you are
  wrong, except you.
- Self-awareness is crucial. 'Awareness is the number-one
  place that I start with all of my clients. I have worked
  with hundreds and hundreds, if not thousands, of
  business owners – and with my children: getting them to
  see that there's a link between that internal narrative and
  the physical manifestation of it. You can give ten people
  exactly the same strategy and say, "Do this A, B, C, D,
  E, go", but it's always down to their mindset. When we
  can understand that, the changes are unreal.'
- But in midlife, isn't it hard to change behaviours? We
  get stuck in a rut – physically and often mentally, don't
  we? 'I think this is the biggest problem. A lot of people
  that come to work with me in their forties and their

fifties, they say, "Oh, that's it. There's no chance for me. I am who I am. I can't change it." I say to them, "Well, with that attitude to start off with, you won't change anything." But then I explain to them there's a whole new area of science called neuroplasticity which shows us that we can actually change our brains through repetition – it's how we learn as children – and through repetition we can unlearn what we do as adults. It comes from understanding why you are the way that you are and the conditioning that led you to be the person you are ... then looking at ways to change. That doesn't happen overnight, but you start to put those building blocks, start to change the words that you use around everything you do. Think about repeating a positive mantra in the mirror every day, and note how you feel after a week when you say it. You might feel silly at first – saying, "I believe today is going to be a good day" at your reflection, but after a week, you might find you look forward to saying – and believing – it.'

- Never forget that words are powerful. 'You say to yourself, I'm never going to change; I'm never going to win; I'm never going to have success; you are creating your future. It takes discipline and commitment to change what goes on up here (in your head), especially after decades of being the person that you have been, but it can be that simple – just to think about words.'

The Midpointer View

DJ extraordinaire Edith Bowman has maintained her midlife mental health by working out what makes her feel good – and doing more of it. Successfully navigating

The Midpoint to her means being 'more aware of myself and what I put into my body, and what I do to nourish my body. If I've got twenty minutes, I'll jump on the bike because I really feel now, more than ever, the benefits of exercise. A bit of Peloton, a bit of yoga, a bit of wild swimming – which I love. I think realising what makes me feel good is the kind of thing that I need to be paying attention to.' But if you feel a crisis coming on, what can you do? 'You don't know how you're going to feel tomorrow, you might wake up in a funk or with a fog. Just recognising that and going, All right, it's going to be one of those days and I'm going to get through it because you go to bed, and tomorrow's going to be another day.'

THE ART OF CHILLING OUT

Dr Nerina Ramlakhan helps us to understand how to switch off, get rest, appreciate the present moment and not worry too much about the future – crucial when safeguarding your mental health. In her book *Tired but Wired*, she shares ideas to maintain well-being when life gets sad, mad or bad. She learnt these skills the hard way – through personal experience. 'I once had huge problems being able to be in the moment. Everything was going so fast. The world is so speedy and a lot of this is to do with technology and the way we've responded to it. We're constantly putting our attention out there but in order to sleep well and to sleep deeply and restoratively, we need to be here right now in our bodies.'

But living in the moment is hard to do when you're a midlifer, constantly asking yourself questions and mulling over every decision you've ever made. 'It's a profoundly questioning time and I can certainly relate to that myself. There's a reason why we call it the sandwich years because there'll be hormonal changes and physiology changes, which makes you more vulnerable to having sleep problems. Your nervous system changes and we need to know how to adapt. I have used my personal insight, my professional experience, my background and physiology, my experience of working with so many people over the years to find really practical ways of stilling themselves, finding their balance point when there's a storm going on around them, stilling the nervous system, helping them to understand what's going on in the nervous system and to navigate from running in survival mode – which is the sympathetic nervous system – into the safety mode – which is the parasympathetic. I start with something called the five non-negotiables, which are the five things that will reset the nervous system if you do them for seven to twenty-one days. And then once we've applied the five non-negotiables, we've reset the nervous system and cleaned up the energy a bit, we can start to go deeper.'

Often, Nerina explains, that's when you'll start to work with the real source of the sleep problem, or your low mood or anxiety. 'The reason why the person can't slow down is because they're running on fear. Why? Maybe it's the relationship that doesn't feel good and they don't want to address it, or maybe it's the job that they're in, they've got a jackass of a boss or something, but they haven't got the resources to deal with it. But once I help them to find their resources with those five non-negotiables, they're then ready to deal with the source of the problem.'

NERINA'S FIVE NON-NEGOTIABLES FOR BETTER MENTAL WELL-BEING

1. If you're waking up with anxiety, if you're having difficulty getting to sleep or staying asleep, if you've got that knotted feeling in the pit of your stomach, as soon as you wake up and your mind is racing, don't

fast. Eat breakfast within about forty-five minutes of rising and include in that breakfast a source of protein. Eat, don't skip breakfast.

2. Don't use caffeine as a substitute for food. It's going to rev up the sympathetic nervous system and you'll continue to run in survival mode.

3. Hydrate your body and ideally alkalise some of that water so that your cells soak up the liquid, your brain soaks it up and your sleep biochemistry works optimally.

4. Get to bed earlier, at least three or four nights a week. The 'architecture' of our sleep is intelligent and the sleep before midnight sets you up for amazing deep sleep as you go. It sets the rhythm of your sleep throughout the night. It's like doing a good warm-up before a game, and it also helps to detoxify the brain. It reduces coronary risks. (More on the power of sleep later.)

5. Get your phone out of the bedroom. Cultivate a healthier relationship with technology when you wake up during the night. Everyone wakes up during the night, it's normal. Don't look at the time. Don't pressurise yourself to sleep. Don't look at your phone. Find your restfulness in your body, feel your way back into your body. Put one hand on your belly, put one hand on your heart, notice your breathing, and drop down into rest. Think about resting.

HAPPY FEET

Piers Morgan and I have something in common: we both love going on long walks to boost our mood and improve our mental health. 'I find however bad the conditions are, apart from torrential rain, going for a two- or three-mile walk really does clear my head and I need it,' Piers shared with me. 'I write lots of columns. I probably pump out three to four thousand words a week on top of all the television stuff, and you've got to be mentally alert to write good columns. It can take me twice as long to write a good column if I'm feeling tired and lethargic as it does when I'm feeling on it. And I actually find just walking at a brisk pace in fresh air, even if it's not sunny, in fact particularly if it's cold, clears the head in a way little else can.'

I agree. I love a cold, brisk walk – I've been known to walk up to three hours sometimes, which my kids can't get their head around, and for a while became a bit of a walking obsessive actually.

Taking as little as twenty minutes out of your day to take a walk outside gives you a long list of benefits needed to boldly navigate the midlife:

- Calms the nervous system, blood pressure and heart rate
- Improves sleep, focus and attention span
- Strengthens the immune system
- Increases vitality, energy, brain power and clarity of thought (as noticed by Piers)
- Restores feelings of awe and gratitude as you observe the changing weather and seasons

The Midpoint View

Witty and wonderful Mariella Frostrup has found that the wisdom – and sense of reality – she's accumulated over the decades has really helped her stay mentally healthy through the midlife years. 'There are benefits to growing older definitely, but ... you need to seek them out. But one of them most definitely that I think we

should all point to is that sense of knowing yourself –
and not in a ranty, angry, old women way, but in a way
where you feel like whatever the fallout is, it's worth it
because you know what you think and you see no reason
not to expect it.'

SAFEGUARDING OUR MIDLIFE MENTAL HEALTH

Life Coach Simon Alexander Ong, author of *Energize: Make the
Most of Every Moment*, has a lot to teach us about looking after
ourselves mentally and physically at the halfway stage. There's this
perfect confluence, isn't there, of children getting older, parents
getting older and other relationships being under a lot of strain
for other reasons, whether it's due to health or financial problems,
and our energy dissipates and our drive to fulfil our own goals
dwindles. It feels like we were given a pot of energy when we
were born, and we've used it all up. I wanted to find out from
Simon what his tips were for looking after our mental health in
these often-exhausting years. Often, he says, it does mean putting
yourself first.

We must understand how to say no gracefully. We can be so
afraid to say no. We worry we're letting someone down and not
living up to our obligations. But we can't really help others until
we help ourselves. It's like the analogy of the aeroplane. When you
board a plane, you have this security briefing and the air stewards
remind us that in case of an emergency, put your own oxygen
mask on first before helping others. Why? Because if we attend to
ourselves first, we can then help as many people as we want. And
that's why it's important to learn we can say no in a graceful way
that shows respect and kindness. Keep in mind that everything
we say yes to means we are having to say no to something else.

And the question is, are you saying no to the very thing that can actually help you move forward and serve you in where you want to be? If we are giving our energy away to everything and everyone, eventually we're going to burn out. And so, we do have to have some sort of balance, and how that balance looks for each of us will be different depending on our circumstances and our lifestyle.

Simon also advises taking a step back to think and rest. 'There is wisdom in silence. Silence is far from empty. It is full of answers. Meditation is powerful and there's a reason why so many people champion this activity because not only does it help us to understand ourselves better, but it grounds us in the present moment.'

MIDPOINT ACTION POINTS

- Never feel embarrassed or ashamed if you're feeling low, anxious or depressed. Seek help from friends and family who can help, and/or your GP.
- Escape the noise for a bit. The hamster wheel we have placed ourselves on might not work for us any more as we get older. You don't have to be stressed to be successful. Start saying no and listening to your own needs. You only have bandwidth for so much, so block time in your life for rest, recuperation and quiet time if you need it.
- If you feel yourself spiralling, remember the things you can control: your thoughts, your actions, your words, your behaviour, how you spend your free time.
- Focus on things that boost happy endorphins and reduce stressful cortisol: journalling, cycling, walking, spending time in nature, taking a cold dip, or having a kitchen disco.

PART TWO

What is happening in our bodies?

4 FITNESS

Start where you are. Use what you have. Do what you can.

ARTHUR ASHE

You may have noticed I am a fan of exercise. In an ideal world I will do something every day, even if it's only a long brisk walk. I am always a better, happier person for a bit of movement. Mental wellness and exercise are inextricably linked whatever stage of your life you're in but as we get older exercise becomes even more vital. Every academic study that has ever been undertaken on growing old has pointed to physical fitness as one of the most important pillars of ageing successfully. And I like the term 'ageing successfully' because I can't understand why you'd want to get older unsuccessfully – which for me would mean not retaining the physical ability to do things. Anyone can just get older (apart from those who don't), but I want to be able to go on long bike rides, play tennis with my (imaginary) grandchildren, dance the night away at a party, be able to walk up Munros and mountains in my seventies and lead as independent a life as is possible into my old age. If I can do that, and have some control over it, the idea of getting older doesn't scare me half as much.

In my teens I was a high-performing gymnast so training for three hours a day was the norm. In my twenties I saw exercise as a way to burn calories and mainly just ran around the block until

I felt I had burned enough of them. In my thirties I wanted to challenge myself and discovered weight training and yoga, but I was still in the mindset that exercise was a way of losing weight, something magazines told us we should all aim for no matter what the scales showed us.

Then in my forties a shift happened. Realising I was never going to be a Vogue-sized, skinny-thighed supermodel, I started to love the body I had been given and knew I wanted to look after it. Nowadays, I look at more than just the number on the scales. I want to be strong enough to move furniture, have endurance to dance the night away at a party and be supple enough to pick things up from the floor without having to bend my knees and okay, I want to carry on doing the splits – it's a pretty good party trick if nothing else.

If you are reading my love letter to exercise thinking, *It's too late for me, no chance, I haven't run since Year 10 PE, I am never going to enjoy it*, please don't give up on yourself. It has become clear from research that you are never too old to start or for it to make a positive impact on your life expectancy and quality of life. This might sound obvious but if you haven't been brought up with sport or fitness, the language and habits around it can be off-putting and you may well decide, I have got this far without it so why start now?

Here's why . . .

- It is a fact that if you don't exercise your rate of physical and mental decline will be quicker than someone who does, even if you have similar diet and other lifestyle factors. I have tried hard to seek out experts on *The Midpoint* who have positive takes to impart to those who have been reluctant exercisers in the past, to find ways to initiate the new or nervous into my exercising love fest. This chapter will contain some of those learnings which are too important to ignore.

- Your motivation to exercise might be to maintain a good weight so your clothes feel nice, to be able to stay at the same pace as your partner on a bike ride or to run a marathon, but whatever level you are at what you will achieve as a by-product is a better chance of warding off disease and illness. And *not* getting sick is definitely something that motivates me to exercise. I want a robust immune system and I know that if I do succumb to any seasonal bugs or flu my body has a better chance of beating them if it's fit.

- We know exercise improves your immune system and we don't need to be training for a marathon to see the benefits. A 2017 study conducted at the University of California San Diego School of Medicine found that just twenty minutes of moderate exercise every day was sufficient to stimulate the immune system, producing a beneficial anti-inflammatory response in the body, which would reduce the risk of arthritis, fibromyalgia and conditions related to obesity.

- Midlifers often complain of being tired, of not getting good quality sleep, of waking up a lot in the night ... Another benefit of working out is it helps increase energy levels during the day and deepens your sleep at night, especially if you are exercising outdoors. I could never work out when I was younger how I could feel exhausted just before a training session and then totally wired and pumped after it. First the endorphins (hormones) released when you exercise make you feel great and activate the happy side of your brain so you will just feel more positive about pretty much everything. Even a quick walk for ten minutes will energise you if you are having an afternoon energy slump.

- Then there is the longer-term effect of helping to boost oxygen circulation inside your body. This happens because exertion helps produce more mitochondria inside your muscles' cells (these are the powerhouses of cells, creating fuel out of glucose from your food and oxygen from the air you breathe). Put simply, more mitochondria equals more energy. Which is why people often find they get a burst of energy after they have exercised.

MORE IS MORE

Greg Whyte, the sports scientist who I introduced earlier, has been on *The Midpoint* a lot and one of the messages he leaves listeners with every single time is that as we get older, we need to do more not less. This idea of slowing down as you age should not be applied to exercise. His mantra is: 'You have to work harder as you get older.' Greg is in his late fifties and recently swam the length of the Thames, so he's walking the walk – or swimming the swim, so to speak.

'The first thing to think about is the myth in society that as we get older, we can start taking it easy,' says Greg. 'That is utterly erroneous. It's absolutely the complete antithesis of what we should be doing. As we age, what we should be doing is working harder. What we have sadly – men and women – is this inexorable decline in physical capacity. We lose muscle mass, a process called sarcopenia. We lose aerobic capacity and effectively performance starts to drop off. But with the right intervention, with the right exercise, with the right approach, we can offset that. It is inexorable, it will happen. But look at some athletes in their fifties, sixties and seventies who are still smashing out performances. They're not as quick as they once were when they were thirty, but nonetheless, what they've done is they've slowed that inexorable decline. But that only comes about by working harder than you did when you were a kid.'

IS MY HEART IN IT?

I like to train to my heart rate when I am doing an HIIT or cardio session, so running, cycling or any kind of jumping around. I use wearable tech (a watch which reads my heart rate or a heart rate monitor) to tell me the level I am working at. Before you start training, find out what your resting heart rate is. The rate you work to is personal, but you can work out what your maximum effort or 10/10 is by going as hard as you can on a bike for a minute, to the point you can't go any harder and you are puffing and red. Then look at what level your heart rate is. Whatever that number is (for example it might be 175bpm) you should think of it as 100 per cent of your max effort, then think about working towards 80 per cent of that for a steady run or ride of half an hour or forty-five minutes, or you might do quicker intervals with a rest that take you to 90 per cent of your maximum heart rate. It's very much your journey; work to your capacity.

The Midpointer View

Andrew Cotter knows it's hard to keep exercising, but it must be done. 'Perversely, when your body is less capable of it, that's when you should be doing more and more exercise. It's like an ever-decreasing triathlon [situation] as you get older, because eventually you'll lose running, then you'll lose cycling, until eventually you'll just be paddling around in a pool in your eighties. But you've got to keep trying to do something. That's the key thing. That's why I really, really dislike seeing people who have healthy, young bodies not taking care of them because what a privilege it is to have that body and just waste it. They'll maybe regret that in later life. But while you've got it, use it, for God's sake.'

MUSCLE MANIA

Muscle is our friend. The more muscle we have the quicker we burn calories, even when we are resting, and muscle is what will keep our frame upright and give us a good posture. But we need to work harder to retain muscle as we age because sarcopenia – the loss of muscle mass due to ageing – speeds up as we leave our twenties. From the age of thirty you are already losing 3–5 per cent per decade and even if you are active, you will still be losing some muscle mass. This is why everyone over the age of forty is recommended to do some resistance or weight training and for women this has the added importance of helping to improve bone density and prevent osteoporosis, which becomes more urgent with the drop-off in hormones after the age of fifty. Don't be afraid of weights. As a midlife man or woman, you are not going to become muscle bound unless you decide to embark on a very high-protein diet, train for hours a day with very heavy weights, and perhaps take some human growth hormone. For most of us, a few hours a week will just about help to retain the muscle we have.

I spoke to Mel Deane, a trainer and ex rugby player, about the importance of strength training and he shared some of the plus points of picking up weights in the midlife. 'The benefits are improved bone density and improved heart health. If you get some more muscle mass on you, you are going to burn more calories, then you're going to burn the fat. There's no downside to it, unless people's posture when they're lifting is incorrect, so I'm a bit of a stickler for that. I'll say, "When you're putting that weight down, don't drop it, put it down as carefully as you pick it up. Imagine there is a rope out of the top of your head, your shoulders are back." People say, "But I don't stand like that." Right? But if you accentuate it when you're doing some lifting, and your spine is in line, you're as strong as steel, head to heels. Be dead straight. This helps in general with posture, too. Everybody needs to be that bit more upright. And people should aim for two strength-training sessions per week.'

I asked Mel for his most important exercise to improve posture and he told me about something called the Sky Dive. 'Lie on the floor with your spine in a straight line, then take your chest off the floor, then take your legs off the floor. You basically look like an inverted banana, or a skydiver in mid-air, and you're firing up all those muscles in your shoulders and your erect back. Hold for a few seconds and then repeat ten times. When you stand up, think about maintaining that position, and that would be a perfect posture. Get used to firing up those muscles, and your posture will improve day to day.' You could be doing that every morning when you wake up.

SETTING GOALS

Having a goal is a good idea and when I started being a bit more serious about weights a few years ago I set about trying to improve my pull-ups and got enormous satisfaction when I managed to get up to six, the number I'd set myself as a challenge. However small the goal feels, it will help focus your training and make it more purposeful.

I look at the week ahead on a Sunday evening and think about what I can fit in, and even if I am exercising on my own, I will pop the time I intend to exercise into my diary so I have already committed that appointment to myself – whether it's a run, a class or a dog walk. Have a think about what movement you could incorporate into your week that you could stick to and write it down – even if you just set yourself the challenge to dance along to the radio for twenty minutes every morning.

So, you say you're time poor? If you've only got two minutes, do a bit of plank. You could do it watching telly or while you're waiting for the kettle to boil, start with thirty seconds then build up. You can do it pretty much anywhere, can't you? It's a great core strengthener and anything is better than nothing. (Remember good technique, pull your belly button up and don't raise your bum, it's called a plank for a reason.) If you hate the plank, do ten burpees. And if you have no idea what I'm talking about, get on the internet. There are so many great apps which offer exercise programmes or advice to inspire you to start a whole myriad of ways to stay or get fit.

NEVER GIVE UP, NEVER SLOW DOWN

Back to Olympian and ultra-athlete Greg Whyte, challenge trainer to people like John Bishop and Davina McCall. He has taught us a lot about how you have to step up your exercise regime in midlife; that you have to do more than you think you need. But it's not all tough news to hear: it doesn't have to be about big bursts of speed; it's about building and strengthening – and keeping it simple if that keeps you on track.

'We call it linear endurance, and it's just repetition. The reason the Couch to 5K programme has been so successful is because actually it's simple. Cycling is simple, too. You get on a bike and you push the pedals around and you move forward; it's instantly rewarding and you get a view that you wouldn't normally get if you were in your car. To run or cycle, you don't have to have expensive equipment, although there are fun, more pricey toys to buy if you want to – trainers, bikes etc. These sports are the perfect confluence of midlife, where you may have a bit more time and money at your disposal because the kids are older.'

I get that: both cycling and golf took a back seat for about a decade when my kids were smaller because I couldn't justify the time they took. I felt I needed to be out for a couple of hours for a decent bike ride, and a round of golf is never less than four hours. Now the kids have left school I have dusted down both bike and clubs and I am enjoying the skills and fitness challenges they pose.

Greg's tips for keeping up the drive and
love of exercise at The Midpoint

I asked him about the most effective kind of training. If you're only going to do one thing, if you're reading this and thinking, Okay, I'm forty-four, I'm seeing where my strength's going and my conditioning, what should I do? What's the best use of my time? Here are his answers.

- The simplest answer is to do what you enjoy. I think that's really important because if you do what you enjoy, you'll do it for longer, you will work harder at it and you'll keep doing it. Far too many times, I speak to clients of mine who say, 'Next year I want to run the London Marathon.' The first question I ask them is, 'Do you like running?' And many of them say, 'No, I hate it.' But it's like this social thing that if you are going to do something, you've got to run the London Marathon! Think critically: you've got do what you enjoy, what you love and what you're passionate about. That makes all the difference in keeping going.
- Strength is one of the most critical factors as we age. We do lose muscle mass; men at a more accelerated rate than women, particularly as they move into their mid-thirties and beyond. And with that loss of muscle mass comes loss of strength, loss of power – those things that underpin performance and help us to avoid injury.
- We know that exercise is crucial in increasing growth hormone secretion, and the higher intensity of the workout, the greater the growth hormone secretion, i.e. helping to keep that powerful testosterone circulating. Remember, testosterone is a sex hormone that helps to regulate bone mass, fat distribution and muscle mass – it's not just about libido. So again, it points towards

this issue of working harder as we get older. And we shouldn't be afraid of actually pushing ourselves. I think sometimes as we age, we sort of think perhaps we shouldn't go that hard. We shouldn't lift that much. We shouldn't go that fast, when actually, as long as everything else is well, as long as we are in good health and we have no underlying conditions, we can push ourselves as hard as we ever did. That doesn't mean to say that it'll be the same power output at the same speed, but we should be pushing ourselves from what we call a perception of effort. We should be pushing ourselves as hard as we possibly can as we age. And that will help counter those changes in specific hormones as well as other factors.

- If you have a healthy cardiovascular system, you really can't push yourself too hard. But if you mentally try to gauge 8–9/10 for effort you'll be near where you should be. Activity is along a spectrum. At one end of that spectrum is sedentism, at the other end of that spectrum is the super-elite athlete. And I think there is good evidence that actually with athletes, they can push it too hard. They can do too much fundamentally linked to under-recovery and under-fuelling, which can lead to all sorts of problems. But for most of us in the general population spending an hour in the gym, we should not be in danger of pushing too hard.

- Think about what you're trying to achieve from that session. Certainly, what we do know – and we did some lovely studies back in the nineties on this – is if you exercise in the morning, it can feel more difficult. So, find the right time for you. If you're feeling tired and try to do a Peloton session, for example, it is going to feel so much harder than if you're in a wakeful state where you're fully energised. There's a lot of psychology in there, not just physiology. Often, it's better to leave a high-intensity workout until you are ready for it, until you are up for it, until you are fully energised. In the morning, something like a moderate-intensity activity like lifting weights or Pilates might work better.

- It's hard to stay motivated in the wintertime. Short days, poor light, rain – they play with you psychologically. They just make it a little bit more miserable, particularly if you're not really up for exercise. Pick something you love at those times when you're feeling a little bit low in energy and can't really be bothered. The last thing you want to do is push yourself to do something that you don't enjoy, because you won't maintain it.

HOW EXERCISE CAN AGE PROOF YOUR BODY

The research done by exercise physiologist Dr Peter Herbert into working out – especially for midlifers – shows that if we can keep moving, we can halt ageing from a cardiovascular standpoint, and even sometimes reverse it. 'The evidence is indisputable, showing how effective high-intensity interval training is in improving our aerobic capacity. In 2012, I conducted a study to investigate the effects of HIIT training on fit and unfit men aged between fifty-five and seventy-seven, who followed a six-week programme of exercise. We found, with all the participants, a small amount of training could have a huge impact, and improvements in aerobic fitness are going to give everyone a much better quality of life. We absolutely showed this study because it could convince sedentary people that they can decrease their risk of morbidity, lower the chances of getting diabetes, lower the chances of getting cardiac problems, and reduce their cholesterol, with some high-intensity exercise.'

Dr Herbert's tips for getting the sedentary on the move

- You need to include aerobic exercise (walking, jogging, running, swimming, etc.) and resistance training (weights, or lifting shopping bags, i.e. finding ways to use your muscles when doing the housework).
- Find an activity you enjoy. Exercising outdoors can be particularly beneficial if you love nature, or you can meet up with a friend, take part with your family, etc.
- Start slowly, then build up. Don't scare or injure yourself by doing too much. Begin with just a few minutes, gradually increasing the time or speed later on. Light exercise is better than no exercise at all.

The Midpointer View

Bestselling author Jane Fallon enjoys working out because it reminds her she is still strong, physically and mentally. 'You get to that stage where you realise you've got to work out a lot more than you ever did to be in slightly worse shape than you ever were before. I enjoy being older but it is all falling apart a bit. I started [working out] because it made me feel better about myself. The mental health side of it kicks in and I really enjoy seeing what I can make my body do. I was a sporty child and teen, but lost it a bit in my thirties and forties. I did find it when I hit my fifties, when I hit that phase where suddenly you think, Oh, everything's going to go a bit south. The thing that got me back into it was I tried to do a cartwheel somewhere in my late forties and I was too scared, I couldn't do it. And I thought, I'm way too young to be too scared to do that and feel like I'm not strong enough. So, I took up yoga and that was my first sort of step back into embracing fitness, as opposed to just doing the odd little gym session here and there. So, I did that, obviously got my cartwheel back, and from there, once had I done yoga for a while, I realised it was easy to start running. I completely organise my whole life around [exercise now]. Every time I put things in my diary, I'm thinking, Okay, so what time can I work out that day? Just because I know I'm going to want to, even if sometimes I wake up in the morning and think, Oh, I don't know if I can face it today! But I would never cancel my trainer because I know the second I start, I'm going to absolutely love it. I wish I'd had that realisation earlier on because the one thing I haven't managed to get back is my flexibility. I'm nowhere near as supple as I was.'

WOMEN ON THE MOVE

Kate Rowe-Ham, who runs the online community Own Your Menopause, is a coach who focuses on diet and exercise for midlife women. 'It's a time that we need to look after our bones, our muscles, our brains, our mental health,' she says, advocating for women in this demographic to find new exercise routines that work for them. Kate suggests finding exercises that work not only for your body but for your brain. 'We've been so surrounded by HIIT and all these really strenuous workouts, which massively raise our cortisol levels at a time when we're already quite stressed, juggling family life, kids, elderly parents. It's really important that we just take a step back.'

For midlife women, she loves strength training. 'Historically, there's been this perception from a lot of women that if they do weights, they're going to really bulk up. In the midlife, your chances of that – unless you're injecting yourself with steroids – are absolutely zero. It's important to lift weights because when our oestrogen depletes, it gets harder to build muscle, which has a negative impact on our bones as well. So, eating a lovely high-protein diet and lifting weights helps.'

But what about those aches and pains, which get more frequent when we hit a certain age, and put us off exercising? Remember some of these niggles can come from being sedentary and inflexible, so exercise can help alleviate them. Listen to your body. But when they are worse than that? 'Be kind to yourself. We may feel pressure to continue to train when we have pain, but we shouldn't. Look at walking, yoga or Pilates or stripping [your exercise routine] back and making sure that you are building in mobility. But some of the aches and pains may have come from living a life that's too sedentary, a life where you have ignored flexibility. Try to keep moving every day, even if you do have slight pain, because we need to keep those joints mobile. Often, I think when we do ache, we think the best thing is to not move but something is always better than nothing, even if it's just that mental gain from feeling that you've done something. Walking is so underrated. There's nothing like a good walk to get that heart rate going. And if you're aching, and if you were my client, I'd also ask you to taper back on gluten, dairy, alcohol and sugar, which all cause a lot of inflammation in the body. All these weird things creep in when we hit midlife that we'd been fine with before. Suddenly, we hit that magic forty and fifty years, and things begin to escalate.'

MIDPOINT ACTION POINTS

- Don't give up too easily or because you're bored. Keep trying things out until you hit upon the exercise that makes you feel good and that you are going to stick to: join a running club so you have others to keep you accountable, a dance class, hike with your family, take the dog on extra-long walks. Do what feels good for your mental and physical health, and ask your GP before starting any new intense workouts.

- Even a little tweak can benefit you in the long term. Dr Peter Herbert's study was based on a very small amount of training, just three very intense minutes of cardio every five days. It's important to know that the men were all of a basic level of fitness at the start of the six-week trial but the effects of the study in terms of cardiovascular health lasted for four years. Start small and you can only grow.
- As comedian John Bishop reminds us, 'The only thing that will stop you doing it is your mind. You've got to train your mind to know that this is just something you do. And the longer it gets used to you just babbling along, jogging, you'll finish it.' I know it's easy to say it's all in the mind, but if there's one thing I have learnt from the elite athletes I have met over the years it's that their minds are way more powerful than any of their pecs, abs or glutes.

5 NUTRITION

One cannot think well, love well, sleep well, if one has not dined well.

VIRGINIA WOOLF

'Let thy food be thy medicine and medicine be thy food' said Hippocrates over 2,400 years ago, his idea being that nutrition is the most important tool in preventing and curing disease. I am a big advocate of proactive health; taking ownership appeals to my inner control freak, and food is where it all starts for me.

My family think I am a little obsessed with what we put in our mouths every day. I see their eyes glaze over when I regale them with scientific facts and statistics about why we are eating lentils or wild salmon for dinner. Even though my husband is gluten-intolerant and was a professional sportsman who watched his diet, it was having our kids which really changed our culinary and nutritional focus. 'Why has everyone else got sweets in their treat drawer but we have rice cakes?' my son Reuben asked me when he started going to other houses on playdates. I know, I know . . . I was *that* mum.

But I stuck to my guns on trying to, all but, eliminate sugar having read that the World Health Organization as early as the mid 2000s was so concerned about the global tsunami of health issues that were coming because of the effect of high sugar diets across the planet, it suggested we should have a maximum of two sugary treats a week, and by that it meant the equivalent of two biscuits. Let's just stress that, the WHO was suggesting two biscuits a week, not a day. I grew up in a house where a packet of biscuits lasted barely an hour once my mum had unpacked the shopping. Sugary foods, in our society, are viewed as an easy comfort. We were never going to be able to police sugar intake outside of our home but inside I decided I'd do my best to make sugar a treat and not the norm. Incidentally, my son is now an eighteen-year-old, 6ft 5in, 115kg rugby player. I often joke with him that we didn't do such a bad job after all on rice cakes – although he does still like sugar!

Midlife throws a few curve balls at our diets and dining habits for us to consider, such as the slowing down of our metabolic rate and the changing levels of hormones and how that then affects fat distribution. Then if we don't adhere to the 'move more' philosophy and we don't address increases in stress that we might be experiencing in midlife through a myriad of factors, we will now have a lifestyle which brings us weight gain, plus potential disease and heart health issues.

TRUST YOUR GUT

Somewhere in my forties, my relationship with food shifted into a healthier mental space. I was previously a subliminal calorie counter; I knew if I took more in than I was giving out I would gain weight. But like a lot of Gen Xs, I was also still shaking off the nineties obsession with the Atkins diet. Even if you never tried it, Atkins was everywhere. Atkins, an American cardiologist, had suggested in the 1970s that a diet high in protein and fats but low in carbohydrates was the way to weight loss and heart health, and around a staggering fifty million people worldwide bought his 1990s book, *Dr Atkins' New Diet Revolution*. As a generation who had been brought up thinking pasta was a health food, this book was a mind blower – and of course as a way of eating it worked to a degree: if you don't eat bread and pasta, you cut out a lot of calories and you will lose weight. Years later and into my forties, I started to work with a trainer who was horrified at the lack of carbs in my diet. I didn't even think I was restricting them and he explained why I needed them (mood regulation, energy levels, heart health and digestive health) and how I was actually going to be healthier and leaner by incorporating the right carbs (legumes, beans and whole grains, to name three) at the right time of day.

Good gut health is crucial to a happy, healthy midlife – boosting immunity from illnesses and diseases, regulating hormones and releasing mood-enhancing serotonin. I started to look at food through the prism of the goodness and the *repair* it was bringing my body, whether it was anti-inflammatory or had healing properties, and above all I became aware of gut health. I'd always been someone who'd have little episodes of bloating and often tried to work out which food it was caused by. Once I started to understand more about the foods that can cause bloating and the ones that help the gut increase the good bacteria in it, and how that all impacted my mood, skin, sleep and energy, I would say it's been one of the most important factors in my diet.

I have a regular bowel movement (sorry I'm not bragging but this is important) and if I don't 'go' for the first time by 10 a.m. I know something isn't right. Although it is important to stress that everyone's 'normal' is different. Pooing is getting rid of excess waste in the body, that's why you feel better and lighter when you have been and the opposite when you haven't. If you feel you aren't going enough or too much then there could be other health issues at play which might mean you need to see a doctor, but if you'd just like to be more regular then a dive into understanding gut health could be a good way forward.

The main ways I've boosted my gut health and keep regular include adding probiotic and fermented foods to my diet, things like natural yogurt, sauerkraut, miso and kimchi – which are now all easily accessible at supermarkets and reduce inflammation in the gut. I also make sure I'm getting enough prebiotic-rich foods, including wholegrains, onion, garlic and bananas, which all boost the beneficial bacteria in my gut.

FAST LOVE

It doesn't work for everyone, but fasting has also become a really hot area of growth and debate among the midlife community. There are many different opinions as to how long you should fast and whether you should do it at all. I spoke to Rhiannon Lambert, a leading nutritionist, chart-topping podcast host and author of *The Science of Nutrition, Debunk The Diet Myths and Learn How to Eat Well for Health and Happiness*, who explained to me what most daily fasters are doing is simply cutting calories by restricting the window of eating, which allows the body to tap into fat stores for energy in the periods when food is not abundant. Fasting has worked well for my husband, who was struggling to lose a few midlife pounds, as it suits his lifestyle to restrict food until midday and then close his window at 8 p.m. But it doesn't work for me and I haven't cut out breakfast.

There are many different ways to fast. For example, some people have two days a week of only one meal at lunchtime then eat normally the rest of the week. If you have hit a dead end trying to lose some weight it might be something to consider. I don't like talking about weight per se because I know there are vagaries in muscle and bone density which might affect a healthy weight, but it can often be your most trusted brutally honest measurement of where you are and what you might need to do to feel mentally and physically improved.

'It is a diet in disguise. Fasting isn't for everyone; some people may really benefit from it and others won't,' Rhiannon explained on my podcast. 'The science of fasting studies how our bodies react and change during periods of time-restricted eating. Essentially what we're saying is that over a period of time, the gut may undergo regeneration that it doesn't have time to do normally. Common sense tells us, although robust studies have not been done on humans yet, that if we restrict our calorie intake, as fasting forces you to do, you will lose weight. It all comes down to calories and diet quality, but in some it can trigger disordered eating. Or for some, not eating lunch means they'll overeat at dinner. For others it may be really helpful. They may actually feel better. Their digestion may improve because if you are one of those people that normally sits in front of the TV late at night dipping into the crisps or popcorn, restricted eating means that you can't do that any more and you've got a set time window.'

Rhiannon's top tips for good guts

- It's good to leave a two- to three-hour window of no food before bedtime if you can, because your body's got a lot of digestion to do after you've had a meal. And remember that old saying, because it has a ring of truth to it: breakfast like a king, lunch like a prince, dine like a pauper. You need more energy as the day goes on. You need less as you settle down, and unfortunately, digestion can also heat up the body and you might overheat in the evening. For women, especially during midlife and going through menopause or perimenopause, that's not going to help with hormonal fluctuations you're already experiencing, so it can really help just to bring dinner forward an hour.
- There are snacks that contain the amino acid tryptophan and we know that this special amino acid can convert in the brain to serotonin, which is our happy hormone. Nuts, yogurt, mini bowls of oats with milk mixed in,

bananas. They're the best type of snacks to achieve the happy hormone.

- Keep a food diary. Note how you feel after you eat and then you'll notice the patterns of what suits your body. Remember, our gut health is strongly interlinked with our mood and plant consumption helps.

YOU ARE WHAT YOU EAT

What we eat should *enhance* us – not diminish our health – but that doesn't mean we have to sacrifice taste and enjoyment. Like everything we discuss in this book there is a balance to be struck. I once heard a talk my son was receiving online during lockdown from the nutritionist at his rugby club who had presented the boys with a lot of information about the foods they should be eating and avoiding. Then at the end of it he said, 'We know this isn't always possible and some days you'll find it hard to get the right food so live by the eighty–twenty rule and you should be okay.' He was asking them to stick to the diet at least 80 per cent of the time. I thought that was such a brilliant and measured way to communicate with a group of teenagers and that's not a bad ratio for all of us to aim for once we're a healthy sustainable weight – and maybe even ninety–ten if you are feeling up for the challenge of being a bit more stringent. As with so much in life, it's all about balance.

START EATING RIGHT, SOONER RATHER THAN LATER

One of the best tips Pippa Campbell, a functional nutrition and weight loss practitioner who specialises in midlife women, told me on the podcast was if you are an overweight woman, try to shift any excess weight and create new habits before the perimenopause symptoms kick in because it only gets harder after that. Pippa has written a great book called *Eat Right, Lose Weight* aimed at the midlife woman, with a strict three-week diet which aims to rebalance the way you eat based on what 'type' you are.

'Most of my clients are in their forties and fifties, and many of them say, "My diet has been really good, but all of a sudden, I'm gaining tummy fat. I always used to be slim." I explain to them when you go into perimenopause, hormones go all over the place. Progesterone is actually the first hormone to start dropping, and oestrogen dominance in itself can cause weight gain. Oestrogen is the one that controls insulin, and insulin is what controls how much sugar we can metabolise. Suddenly we can't deal with those carbohydrates we were eating – that piece of toast for breakfast, for example – and it's turning to fat. It's unfair but women of our age really need to cut back on their white starchy carbs and replace them with loads of vegetables. I wouldn't say no carbohydrates, women tend to need some carbohydrates, but switch the toast to sweet potato or wholegrain rice, and try having a protein breakfast. It is trial and error because imagine an orchestra if the violin isn't playing or pulling its weight – it's going to affect the rest of the instruments, and they're going to have to work harder and this is what is happening with hormones.'

Pippa's quick tips for a midlife reset
(her weight-loss programme)

- No snacking is a really good rule to follow because it gives your body a mini fat-burning window and gives your insulin levels the change to calm down.
- Eat protein at every meal because that will help boost weight loss and your mood, and support sleep.
- In the first phase of reset, replace your carbs with vegetables. Aim for 500 grams of vegetables a day. Yes, that sounds like a lot of broccoli but you can easily do

that by having a salad at lunch and then vegetables in the evening. They are powerful antioxidants and brilliant for detoxification. Look at your plate: at any meal, half of it should be covered with vegetables. As you reach the weight you are looking for you can start to bring the good carbs back.

WORKING OUT WHAT WORKS FOR YOU

Davinia Taylor was the actress who had the party lifestyle, the glamorous friends and the almost constant paparazzi presence in her life. When her damaging relationship with alcohol came to an end, her life certainly got healthier in one way, but stopping that addiction didn't leave her feeling as physically well off as she might have hoped; she gained a lot of weight – 60 pounds – and wasn't feeling the best version of herself that she could be. It was only when she really addressed her diet, she found true mental well-being, and she's now using her experiences to help people understand how gut health works in relation to all aspects of an improved life. She shared her inspiring story, and the work that came from it, on the podcast.

'When I gave up alcohol, I started to notice that everything – my emotions, my energy, my foggy brain – was working in direct correlation to certain ingredients that I was consuming on a daily basis. As a population, we've become so used to middle-aged bloat and tiredness, and wading through life, that it's becomes the norm and we all speak the same rhetoric. "Oh, I can't be bothered doing this, I forgot this. I'm stressed, I don't get decent sleep." And it really doesn't have to be that way. Hippocrates said that all disease begins in the gut. Do I want to enjoy this Mr Kipling cake for three seconds, and do I want to be operating on a lower happiness level for the next few hours? Forget about a lifetime on the hips and all that! Who cares what you look like physically if your mood's low? If you feed the brain appropriately, the body follows automatically. The body wants to thrive. It doesn't want to be inflamed or sore. I was so inflamed. I was like a walking bruise. And I felt vulnerable. There was no running in me. There was no chase, there was nothing. I had trained my brain to want more dopamine.

I'm not a saint. I'm from Wigan. I eat pies, bloody hell. That's how I was raised. I don't believe in calorie counting. I think calories do have an impact on our weight, but if you are feeding yourself with calories that have nutritional value, you start eliminating cravings. There's a huge conversation to be had about the perimenopause starting in your thirties – you don't have to wait until your fifties. You're at the busiest time in your life, when you've got kids and you've got family and you've got a career in your thirties, yet you're trying to balance your hormones as well, but you need to consider everything that you are absorbing, particularly if you've got a predisposition in your genetic code that you're not that good at it.

So, I started an investigation into biohacking, which means you're hacking into your own biology. It's taken me ten years of being around Harley Street and reading tens of thousands of papers, but preventative medicine is so much easier than trying to cure chronic disease. [In our culture] we don't prevent, we try and cure and it's never a cure. It's always a Band Aid over a gaping hole. I discovered my diet was making me tired – the hidden sugars, the oils that are put in everything, even health foods, to extend their shelf life and get us addicted. Even if I had nine hours' sleep, I was still exhausted and I had no zest for life, no creativity, and I could just about get to the kitchen to have yet another coffee.'

Davinia Taylor's two biggest takeaways

- Always read the label. Forget about what's on the front of a food package, and if it says *free from* be on high alert because free from fat often means higher sugar. Free from gluten normally means higher sugar. Learn what vegetable oils are in your foods and try to take them out. That's super easy. You just turn the label around. If it's got rape seed or sunflower oil, put it back. There are loads more companies out there using avocado oil and olive oil in their ingredients. Your body understands that. It can metabolise it, use it and get it out. It doesn't know what to do with the other two. Even a burger or a sausage, half the time it's got wheat and gluten in, and that could inflame your gut. And when your gut's inflamed, you're not going to make enough serotonin, which is your happy hormone that goes up to your brain. It's the gut–brain axis, and it's paramount.

- I would always have activated charcoal knocking around. If you do slip up, it will mop it up and get your gut rebalanced. It's really absorbent and you can get it from a health food store for next to nothing. Take two of those before and after a takeaway.

VEGGIE OPTIONS

Eat the rainbow – that's the advice we get, regardless of age. But what should middle-aged people be eating more of, I asked nutritionist Nicola Moore. Can we still eat those heavy carb vegetables like potatoes? 'I think potatoes are fine,' she reassured me. 'It's about the balance of how you eat them because when we transition through the menopause, as our oestrogen levels start to decline, our response to another hormone called insulin changes slightly and one of insulin's roles is to help us store fat. That's why we might see weight gain, especially around the middle, and that's not good for long-term health outcomes. So, managing the amount of carbohydrates you eat can be extremely helpful. So have potatoes, but I would say watch the number that you have and make sure you have protein with them. A steak and chips with a lovely great big salad on the side is a good option. Having fish a few times a week is great. Meat, if you like meat or animal-based foods, can give you a very good, easy access to a protein source but vegetarian and vegan sources of protein are also really useful, for example tofu and quinoa.'

The Midpointer View

Nihal Arthanayake, the former rapper and broadcaster, has changed his eating habits so history doesn't repeat itself. 'My dad died of a heart attack at sixty-two, and he told me a few years before that his plan was to get to sixty-five, spend six months a year in Sri Lanka, six months in the UK consulting, and he never got to see it. About six months ago, I had some blood tests and they showed that cholesterol was heading in the wrong direction for type 2 diabetes. I was also discovering that I couldn't go and kick a ball around with my son because I'd be out of breath. I'd put on weight, too, comfort eating during lockdown. All of these things converged on me and I made a decision that I would seriously try and change what I ate and to exercise more. I have to take this shit seriously because if I look after myself in my fifties, then my sixties and my seventies will be much better, but if I don't ... my sixties and seventies are going to be crap, and I'm going to end up looking like Steptoe and I don't want that to happen to me. I'm trying to stay away from white bread and cakes. I can't have cakes in the house, because if I do, I'll eat them all, day to night. I got a very expensive gym membership – and I say that not to boast, I say it because all the cheap ones I'd ever had, I never went because it's easy not to use them; whereas this one hurts me every time that direct debit comes out of my bank account. I sit on a recumbent bike and I cycle my ass off for half an hour and then I swim.'

SWEET ENOUGH?

In recent times, we've been led to believe that sugar is the enemy of midlifers, so I asked Rhiannon Lambert for the lowdown on the sweet stuff. 'There's a lot of myths surrounding sugar. Sugar isn't necessarily "addictive", this is a strong word for it. It does, however, light up reward centres in the brain, which is the reason some people may always have room for more. It's got that feel-good factor and there's a lot of psychological beliefs and behaviours that we've created over the years around sugar. If you think back to your childhood or anything that makes us feel good, there's a common inclination ingrained within us to turn to sugar when we need a pick-me-up. When we're younger, our metabolisms are faster and we haven't started to lose any muscle mass so we are able to process sugars more efficiently.'

But sadly, sugar does become more of a problem as we age. 'If you take a molecule of table sugar by itself, 50 per cent of sugar is fructose and 50 per cent is glucose. Fructose is a fruit sugar. Glucose is the type of sugar we get from carbohydrates. Combine that you've got the white refined sugar. I want to be very clear that we're talking about this white sugar rather than things that come naturally in our foods. That's the stuff we need to be limiting because our consumption is too high in the UK. Now, the reason it's a problem is because first of all, anything that contains sugar has a lot of calories, and when we have a lot of sugar, some research suggests it depletes other nutrients like magnesium within our bodies. And the excess energy, the fructose component of the sugar, gets stored around our liver. The reason excess sugar is so bad in middle age in particular is weight gain and that it tends to store around the areas that we know put you at a high risk of cardiovascular disease. So, I don't want to demonise it because I think sugar has a place within our diets, but we do need to get a balance. Nutritionally speaking, it doesn't offer much to us. That's the thing I will flag. It doesn't offer any benefits to include it within the diet, but then you've got to weigh up your psychological well-being. Try to slowly reduce those extra sugar items you're having; replace them with a natural sugar, like a piece of fruit, rather than having chocolate. If you're going halfway, dip a banana in some chocolate.'

STRESS AND FOOD

We've all heard of having too much stress on our plate? Well, it's not just a saying: what we eat can affect our mood positively or negatively. As we've discussed in earlier chapters, The Midpoint can be a stressful time in anyone's life, balancing a million things and being hit by illness and loss. The good news is you can eat your way calmer. Ruth Wood is a dietician who specialises in mental health and diet, and how they are linked more than we sometimes appreciate. 'The adrenals don't know the difference between a true, horrendous stress or a daily modern stress like sitting in a traffic jam or getting up late and having to rush to work and all those sorts of things, and will release cortisol, which creates an energy surge and cravings for sweet and fatty foods – and fat storage.' Ah, that extra roll around the midriff explained!

'So, in midlife we need to try not to be so stressed, and support our adrenals, blood sugar levels and mood in general by consuming more calcium, magnesium, vitamins B and D, omega 3 and chromium. These nutrients help with mental health, mood and calming anxiety,' says Ruth.

Your new anti-stress shopping list:

Dark green, leafy vegetables, like watercress, spinach and kale
Calcium-rich foods like milk and yogurt
Antioxidant-rich foods like blueberries and oats
Vitamin D-rich foods like eggs
Vitamin B-rich foods like avocados
Zinc-rich foods like oysters, nuts and seeds

MIDPOINT ACTION POINTS

- Midlife is not the time to throw your hands up and give in. By now you've lived long enough that you hopefully have an idea of what good nutrition is even if you don't always stick to it: eating plenty of colourful fruit and vegetables, seeds, nuts and legumes, the best quality meat and fish you can afford, and avoiding ultra-processed food (food containing emulsifiers and other artificial ingredients which you'd never be able to re-create in your own kitchen) as much as possible. Think about signing up to a meal plan, or for a weekly fresh fruit and veg delivery box.
- We often snack and gorge through our twenties and thirties, eating whatever we want with no impact on our weight, and then we get to the midlife and that can change – and we accept it as middle-aged spread. But it doesn't have to be that way. We're not actually meant to suddenly just put on lots of weight! It's often

about *what* we're eating not always the amount, so
think about upping your healthy protein intake and
lowering your starchy carb intake and then watch your
body thank you.

- The good news is it's never too late to eat smarter. A
better diet today will make a difference in the future.

6 AGEING AND BEAUTY

Beautiful young people are accidents of nature ...
beautiful old people are works of art.

ELEANOR ROOSEVELT

If this book was about how to retain youthful beauty then this chapter should probably be read by twenty-year-olds and simply state 'wear a high SPF on your face every day and don't sit in direct sunlight and we'll see you in thirty years'. While I am certainly not a sunbathing fiend (my red-ish Celtic skin doesn't really love it), I won't deny the use of a sunbed in my late teens and early twenties. Actually, even worse than that, I used one before breakfast for a time when we had one in the spare bedroom in the late eighties. I skipped off to school at fifteen years old in my uniform smelling vaguely of burnt flesh. Ah, the eighties; parents were different back then. The damage was probably done before I took my GCSEs, but from my late twenties onwards I tried my best to always use a factor 50 in the hope that somehow it would all balance itself out. The brown spots/large freckles I have on my thighs now would suggest I didn't quite get away with it. There's no use looking back and wishing I had done things differently; all I can do now is look after what I have got.

I have consciously tried to avoid focusing too much on the aesthetic of ageing on *The Midpoint*. I wanted the podcast to focus on the joys and positivity of getting older not the inevitable appearance of more lines, wrinkles and facial sagging, which for most of us appear as the collateral damage of having more birthdays. By the time we get to the midlife we have usually come to terms with the things about our face that might have caused anxiety in our teens and twenties, or we have been lucky enough to have earned enough money to do something about it. And please note, although this is not the book to tell you where the best surgeons reside, I would never judge anyone for deciding that it is the best route for them.

Back to me and my face, then. Regrettably, I spent too much time unhappy with my nose and seriously debated rhinoplasty in my twenties, even visiting a plastic surgeon. I am happy I didn't succumb because I like my large nose now, and as one of my favourite make-up artists says, 'It's your facial scaffolding.' By which I think she means it's holding my skin up for a bit longer, before it sags, than those cute, button noses I coveted when I was younger. The acceptance I now have of my Nubian nose is some proof to me that we do become more comfortable in our skin as we age and I definitely don't covet youthful beauty. Instead, I find myself appreciating a well-groomed woman or handsome bloke closer to my age. I notice the sparkle in the eye of a fifty-three-year-old with a great haircut and an infectious laugh quicker than I would a perfect twenty-year-old with flawless skin . . . because that's what you are supposed to have at twenty as the wise Eleanor Roosevelt mentions above. Which is marvellous for the twenty-year-olds and good luck to them all; they are lovely to behold.

Of course, occasionally I do those things we all do: staring at the rear-view mirror and pulling the skin at the sides of my cheeks back into my ears to see what a facelift would look like when the traffic lights are on red, grabbing the skin at the back of my head to see what a smooth neck would do to my appearance, and I sometimes stare into a magnifying mirror and wonder if my pores are actually bigger than they were or is that my self-tan drops I can see.

If we want to search for imperfections, we can spend all day finding them, but that seems like a very bad use of time to me. And if there's one thing a midlife person knows it's that time is increasingly precious. That's not to say I don't value the time I spend having a facial or sitting in the hairdresser's chair getting my colour done, both of which make me feel fabulous and relaxed, giving a boost to the ego afterwards.

As we age, hair becomes an increasingly thorny topic. On the episode I recorded with broadcasters Jane Garvey and Fi Glover, Jane suggested that the real test of how far women had come in the media would be to see a high-profile broadcaster on TV with grey hair, making the point that there are plenty of men with grey hair but not so many women. Well, it won't be me and that's not because I am in denial, I just don't think it would suit my skin tone and as I have very wavy hair, I'd look like an unkempt ageing poodle, which would be too distracting for the viewers. At the roots I am still a curly mess, with my unruly hair exacerbated by the incoming greys, and in spite of the occasional Brazilian blow-dry – where the technician uses keratin to try to smooth out my mane – I am quite high maintenance when it comes to matters hirsute.

There are reasons for this – it's not just my bad luck. As we age, we produce less oil so the hair becomes less elastic and more brittle; then all the processing so many of us do to our hair – blow-drying, using straighteners and colouring, etc. – makes the condition worse. Having a professional blow-dry is probably the single best thing I do to make me feel I have improved my appearance, it's just a pity that it's adding to the damage which I deal with on a daily basis. I know I have to limit myself to how often I use heat on the hair and keep up with the hair-building treatments ... Short of that working, I have already started googling wigs. Not really. Okay maybe once.

The Midpointer View

I asked television presenter and former model Tess Daly if being known for your looks when you're younger is a factor in how you feel about getting older, and come into midlife. 'I think I've gone the opposite way, because I was judged on what I looked like on the outside,' she said. 'It kind of made me go the other way. I saw that there did not lie happiness on taking someone's opinion of you on board. I saw that it could mess with your sense of self, your well-being. Yes, when you catch yourself in daylight or you look down at your phone, you go, Crikey, what's going on? That's a rude awakening. I was determined, whether subconsciously or not, that I would not let my own happiness rely on how I looked on the outside, because what's the point? It's going to age; it's going to get old and it's going to fall off. It's just a shell. We're a human meat suit walking around. I do believe it's the content of your character, what is inside, that shines out and makes you beautiful. Yes, I've got lines now, but I don't really beat myself up about it. I think, Well what's the alternative? Not being here? So, I'm grateful and happy for a healthy body that's got me this far.' What a great attitude, although she also still looks bloody marvellous.

THE BARE MINIMUM

I believe what I've covered in the two previous chapters probably contributes more to my face and appearance than anything I can do to it topically: nutrition (and good gut health) and fitness, which helps the elimination of toxins, both help to alleviate inflammation, dark circles and lead to a better complexion. Double cleansing (using a cleanser to take my make-up and obvious dirt off the skin and then giving my face a second cleanse to go a bit deeper into the pores and removes bacteria, sweat and old skin cells) and having a good skincare regime have always been in my armoury. I had a few years of nasty break-outs in my early twenties and was troubled with large angry spots in the hormonal area of the face, which is mainly around the chin, so as a result I am fairly religious about how and when I cleanse and moisturise – and it's never too late to adopt a restorative skincare routine.

The menopause does once again play its part for women. It was the increasingly dry skin and dry hair I was experiencing in my late forties which formed part of the picture of symptoms that helped me work out I was perimenopausal. Again, it's falling oestrogen which is to blame; it's the hormone that stimulates the body's production of collagen and oils. I did some work with No7, the skincare range from Boots, after they had undertaken specific re-search into menopausal skin and come up with a range of products tailored to help based on falling ceramides. I am not promoting these products to you specifically, but what I like is that skincare companies are understanding that the midlife woman and man have different needs to their thirty-year-old customer and, in No7's case, were prepared to do research to prove that. The key word in skincare for midlife seems to be ceramides; whatever the brand you are using, ceramides help to build a protective barrier to back up and trap in moisture, and that applies to the body, too – not just the face.

There is no doubt that if you feel good – and for me that is being fit and strong and having a clear complexion – you will radiate something to the outside world that is more powerful than the subjective ideal of 'beauty'. However, nobody on TV at my age rolls out of bed and simply runs a comb through their hair, so as well as exercise and good nutrition these are the must-do things that help me to feel I can put my best foot forward:

- Regular facials and facial massages, which I have learnt to do to myself (Eva Fraser's facial massage book, *Facial Workout*, is a great place to start)
- Eyebrow tint (you can buy good tint online)
- Good skincare regime
- Manicures (I have inherited workers' hands from my mum and grandma)
- Occasional keratin treatments on hair
- Highlights (not ready to go grey yet)
- Tan Luxe drops in my moisturiser to balance my pink skin which doesn't love the sun
- Cold water therapy (swimming and showers)
- Laughter and friendship
- Sex (it really does have benefits for the skin if you need another reason to get your mojo going)

The Midpointer View

Olympian Denise Lewis knows what is really important when it comes to ageing. 'I do not worry about what my face will look like. I look after my skin but what I do worry about is will I be able to do the activities that I enjoy without feeling pain, without the knee flaring up or my Achilles breaking down or my hip giving up on me. I don't really think about what my face is going to look like. I always believe there'll be a cream out there, there'll be make-up out there that can hide a multitude of sins. This is where the athlete kicks in. Do not focus that far into the future, right? Focus on one Olympics at a time.' Having sat next to Denise on the Athletics sofa for the last ten years I can tell you that the woman is flawless so not worrying about her face too much is working.

SKIN DEEP

For a deep dive into how to protect and preserve our skin as we reach The Midpoint, I got Caroline Hirons on the podcast. The woman truly is an encyclopaedia on the subject of not only looking after your skin at this age, but of looking after your attitude too. I asked her if her skin had changed in the last few years – and what she'd done to combat any future issues. She shared that, at around forty-eight, she'd noticed her skin was dry and lifeless, and one of the plus sides to her of going on HRT was that it got her skin back on track. What other tools does she have for maintaining?

Caroline's top tips for a great complexion:

- Be open minded. 'I am a fan of the odd bit of an injectable. When I was sorted with HRT and I started taking care of myself a bit more, I lost weight, and I got more jowly. I went to a friend of mine and said, "Okay, your skin looks amazing, and I know you have the odd tweak. What are you doing?" And they said a teeny bit of filler here. I go once or twice a year. And if someone says, "Oh, what have you had done? You look great", I know it's too much. Whereas if they say, "You look really well", it's like you're wearing a good foundation.'
- Don't paint on your face. 'You want to be wearing the make-up, not the other way around.'
- Help can be found in a jar. 'The gold standard is vitamin A.' Retinoid is your best friend.
- Wear SPF. 'Some people say if the UV factor is low, you don't need to wear an SPF. That might be for UVB, but UVA still shines through and that's what causes your ageing. So, my big thing with my kids is just use your SPF because when you get to my age, you won't have to fix pigmentation damage and things like that. Midlife

women should also still be thinking about wearing it daily – it's never too late to start with your SPF.'

- Go easy on yourself and your skin. 'If you're menopausal, and you over-treat your skin, saying, "I'm going to do acid, then I'm going to do a peel, then I'm going to do some micro-needling ..." Don't. Your skin can't cope. Menopausal women are slower to repair, slower to heal. I always say slow down with the actives. Build up your barrier, which is just using a good solid moisturiser and an SPF, and within a week or two your skin should be back to normal, and then you can look [at what to do next].'

- Collagen can be cool. 'I'm asked all the time about collagen powders and as most of my dietitian and nutritionist friends will say, when you ingest a collagen powder, the stomach doesn't go, "Oh, remember, lads, she wants this in her face." It will be used elsewhere. It'll go to your hair, your nails – so this is no bad thing. But selling people the myth that you can replace lost collagen in the face is just not reality.'

- Lose the booze for better skin. 'The best thing I ever did was stop drinking. I still like the odd glass of champagne, but when you're menopausal, your liver just cannot cope and it shows on your face.'

The Midpointer View

Lorraine Kelly will not be going under the knife anytime soon. 'I'm frightened of plastic surgery. I'm scared of doing things in case it all goes wrong. We've done so many items [on the show] in the past, and poor women have gone for procedures and they end up looking like

Klingons. I mean, it's awful. You don't want to look like someone from *Star Trek*. I think the fear will stop me from doing it. And I think I've earned these lines here. I'll call them laughter lines.'

HOW TO WEAR YOUR HAIR

Michael Douglas, hairdresser (and partner of the wonderful Davina McCall, who as we know, has been an amazing pioneer of the HRT revolution), has become an expert in helping people get their midlife look right. 'My clients, like Dawn French, Kate Bush, obviously Davina, and more – they've all reached this age where they're all going through midlife. It's a hot topic that I never stop talking about or listening about.'

What are the concerns he sees in his salon?

'When you hit a certain age, people find themselves losing hair. As you get older, the cell production of new skin and new hair starts to get worse and worse. I read this scientific paper about how that works. The cell gets reproduced off the previous production of its cells, a bit like a photocopy. So, the first time it gets photocopied it's great, but when you photocopy the photocopy and then photocopy that photocopy, that's essentially how you age. And so, your hair does start to deteriorate because the follicle that produces it just starts to get older. It stops producing colour, so you start to go grey, and then it can start to produce thinner and thinner hair. The menopause has an enormous impact on how well you grow hair. Your hair goes through a growing phase and a shedding phase. About 90 per cent of your hair is in a growing phase, and about 10 per cent is in a shedding phase, and that's when you run your fingers through your hair and pull out some strands. With a drop in oestrogen and progesterone, the growing phase slows down so that 90 per cent of a growing phase turns into about 60 per cent and then you get 40 per cent going into the shedding phase. And that's what people are terrified of. They put their fingers through their hair, and it's falling out left, right and centre.'

So how can we help our hair?

'The slowing down of the growing phase is largely related to hormones, but it's also related to health and diet. People don't eat properly. People just aren't eating enough protein, which is the single best thing you can eat to grow healthy hair. Iron and collagen can be good supplements for healthy hair growth. People give up quite quickly with hair supplements, but stick at it for three to six months.

Do women need to cut our hair short in middle age?

'Your style does not have to change at The Midpoint. You are not too old for long hair. What you want is to just look the best possible version of you. And I often find short hair can emphasise ageing. Don't worry about your face shape. In thirty-five years of doing hair, I've never thought about face shapes at all. It's more what will your hair do and what won't it do? The style has to work for you for the six weeks you are not with me in the salon. Always take pictures to the hairdresser's of cuts you like. Don't ever feel intimidated by that. One of the big problems hairdressers face is not fully understanding what you want, and the best way to break that down is just to show them a picture. And it doesn't matter if it's Jennifer Aniston, it just gives the hairdresser a clear idea.'

The Midpointer View

TV presenter Claudia Winkleman is embracing getting older with a sigh of relief. 'I didn't really like the things you were supposed to do when you were younger, and thank God I don't have to do them any more. I don't like sweating. I don't like movement. I went to yoga, and it smelt of smug and hummus – I couldn't bear it. I don't have to queue to go into a nightclub. I don't have to go to a drinks party and pretend I'm enjoying myself. I don't have to wear tight, sexy outfits. I've been waiting for the moment I can outwardly say, "Do you know what we're going to do this weekend? We're going to do a puzzle and I might make a curry."' But what about ageing? That's not fun, is it? 'We don't have one full-length mirror [in the house] so I've no idea what I look like. But if I stay at places with mirrors, I will often look up and go, "Why is Meatloaf here? I didn't know he was invited."' Although she didn't say it, I think Claudia's acceptance of herself is clear. There are no hang-ups to be found.

LOSING IT

Steve O'Brien is a trichologist who helps people who are losing their hair or having other dramas with their locks in the midlife. Hair loss is the biggest reason people go to him. 'I've been doing this for twenty years. When I started, I would say 90 per cent of our clients were men. In the last five years, it's getting on for 90 per cent women. For women clients I think what is causing hair issues is stress, hormones, and as we're all getting older, circulation is slowing up as well.' I asked him for some easy tips to help hold on to our hair:

- There are a lot of medications that cause problems as well, and a lot of medical conditions – anaemia is a big one – so check your iron levels.
- Women damage their hair with too much blow-drying, straightening, chemical relaxing, braiding. Try to let your hair air-dry more. (I am trying, Steve!)
- Headstands can help boost circulation. (Please don't try this at home unless you are proficient!)
- Argan oil helps the condition of the hair if it's feeling dry, and it has a stimulatory benefit as well.

The Midpointer View

TV presenter and journalist Ben Shephard is feeling his age. 'I'm very conscious of looking a lot more tired than I used to because of early mornings; that catches up with you, for sure. The great thing about the advent of wearing glasses is that you can't see the bags under my eyes. I'm not getting any younger. The thing I am very conscious of is my knees and my back aren't quite what they were. But I certainly am very conscious – I put my neck out the other day wringing out a flannel. I mean, if that's not a proper midpoint … If my teenage self knew I was using a flannel because I had a skincare regime or even just cleaned myself properly, he would be so embarrassed. But the fact that I strained a muscle in my shoulder because I'd wrung it …'

BITE-SIZE INFO ON MIDPOINT TEETH

Teeth go through different stages in your life and the stage I'm at is *can't eat spinach without seeing it stuck later.* I talked to tooth expert Elaine Tilling to ask what's going on in our mouth around the late forties and early fifties. 'Well, the same as what's going on with the rest of the body,' she said. 'Teeth are so much more than just their teeth. If your gums aren't healthy, it links to the rest of your body. The mouth reflects what's going on elsewhere, so it needs a little bit of extra loving care, really like the rest of our bodies.'

What should we be doing for our teeth in midlife?

'Getting your toothbrush right, getting your brushing technique right, using floss, because as we age there are extra nooks and crannies for us to clean. If you're a grinder in your sleep, wear a night guard. The tissue in the mouth ages too, and things are not quite as efficient as they used to be, so the bone will change and bacteria in the mouth causes inflammation, which causes the gums to break down. Teeth do become more porous as we age too, and they love a little bit of red wine and coffee to stain them. Having a regular scale or polish and maintaining your plaque control is key. Your mouth is a bit like a car. I wouldn't expect myself to manage the maintenance of my car, and I don't expect individuals to manage full time the whole of their health. Regular appointments with a dentist and hygienist keep things at bay, and prevention is always better than cure. The earlier we detect signs of disease, the more likely we are to be able to cure it.'

MIDPOINT ACTION POINTS

- Give yourself a head start to looking good by getting the basics down: good sleep, staying hydrated, limiting alcohol and eating food full of vitamins and minerals. It's boring but true.
- Looking after your physical appearance isn't vain – when you look better on the outside, you feel better on the inside, too. It's no one else's business what you do to feel confident and happy with your reflection in the mirror – and likewise, don't judge anyone else either.
- Remember you're still gorgeous. As feminist writer and author of *The Feminine Mystique* Betty Friedan wrote: 'Ageing is not lost youth but a new stage of opportunity and strength.' Don't be depressed when you look in the mirror – there's wisdom in every wrinkle, wit in every line. Embrace your changing beauty, inside and out.

7 SLEEP

Having peace, happiness and healthiness is my definition of beauty. And you can't have any of that without sleep.

BEYONCÉ

Sleep is the most important thing we can do to aid the repair of our body. A bit like good nutrition and a decent skincare regime, you'd hope that once we'd got to midlife knowing that we are happier and healthier when we have a great night's sleep, we'd have found a way to achieve it. And yet it still comes up as one of the most requested areas to keep exploring on the podcast. So why can't we sort out our shut-eye?

Well, those changing midlife hormones can play a huge role in why sleep becomes an issue for us, whether it's struggling to fall off to sleep or waking up after a few hours when we do manage to drift off at bedtime. Fluctuating levels of progesterone and testosterone may affect how you rest, which we'll discuss more in Chapter 9. Here, I want to explore what we can do to hack into our changing sleep patterns before negative habits become embedded, and share some tips I've learnt on catching zzzzzzs.

If you chat to a group of friends about sleep you will get a variety of answers to the question: How do you sleep? The one thing my mates and I can all consistently agree on is that we feel better and operate at a higher level when we have had good sleep. For me, the ideal is around seven hours per night. I can just about handle six and half hours, and if I don't have an alarm I will probably wake naturally after seven and a half hours. What about you? Have you ever noted down your sleeping patterns and your natural wake-up habits? The American Academy of Sleep Medicine has recently given guidelines that seven hours is the magic number for most healthy adults, which was a relief as for a long time I thought I was coming in short and should have been shooting for the fabled eight hours (eight is fine, by the way, but much more and you could be creating issues by having too much sleep, especially if you are still waking up feeling groggy).

If you have an early flight or an alarm call for a special event occasionally, which means you only get about five hours' sleep, you should still be able to function perfectly well as you have enough in the bank. Although if you are anything like me you will be sub-liminally dreading getting up early for days in advance. However, if you consistently only get five hours' or less sleep a night, you run the risk of a range of illnesses and conditions associated with severe sleep deprivation. These include mental, physical and long-term health problems such as:

- Slower thinking
- Reduced attention span
- Poor decision making
- Lack of energy
- Erratic mood changes with a greater propensity to feel stressed or anxious
- Increased blood pressure which can lead to cardiovascular issues
- Obesity and type 2 diabetes

It is for all those reasons we really need to take sleep seriously.

TO SLEEP, PERCHANCE TO DREAM

A lot of couples tell you they don't go to bed on an argument, which Kenny and I also adhere to, but the main reason for that isn't just about repairing the relationship after a petty squabble. No, it's about releasing any tensions and issues from the mind and body. It's virtually impossible to go to sleep when you're jittery or agitated, isn't it? It is not always possible to alleviate all stress before bed – if you have an interview for a job the next day or a long-running situation with work which has caused you anxiety, for example – but what you can do is write a list (mentally or literally) of things that are bothering you in the hours before you go to bed and then throw it away. I have always used lists as a sleep aid. I used to sleep with a pad by my bed so that if something was churning through my mind, I could literally let it go and head off to dreamland. It might not have been a bad thing, even a sudden thought that I had to book the kids a dentist appointment or I hadn't returned a message to someone, but knowing it was on that pad helped my mind to turn off.

RISE AND SHINE

The other day, having seen something on TikTok, my eighteen-year-old daughter Lois informed me she was going to start getting up at 5 a.m. because that's the time most successful people wake up. I told her this was not a new discovery but in fact an age-old trope. When I was young, we were told the same about Prime Minister Margaret Thatcher and how she only needed five hours' sleep a night to run the country. Gen Z has been told to look to Elon Musk as its sleep deprivation poster boy – he says he only needs four and a half hours' sleep, as do a whole host of other billionaire entrepreneurs. Suffice to say, I have no desire to emulate Maggie or Elon. And I warned my daughter: if you want to get up at 5 a.m. you need to be lights out and heading off to sleep by 10 p.m., which for most eighteen-year-olds is the middle of the day. I have a very good friend who gets up at 5 a.m. so she can do an hour of chores and work organisation or half an hour of exercise before any of her four children wakes up. She's disciplined, though, and gets to sleep by 9.30 or 10 p.m. – the only way to rise that early and still give your mind and body enough time to rejuvenate itself.

The key to my friend's successful early rising, and good sleep in general, is consistency of bedtime, something we can all adopt. Getting to bed at the same time and waking up at the same time has been linked to positive sleep health. This is not great news if you are a shift worker whose pattern changes, but for us midlifers who are able to adopt this formula it could be one of the keys to sorting out disturbed sleep. Whatever time you decide to go to bed, try to come off screens for ninety minutes before hand (I know, I know ...), and charge your devices outside of the bedroom if you can (again, I know!) because the blue light emitted by your phone restrains the production of melatonin which controls your circadian rhythm, which regulates your internal body clock. Going old-fashioned and reading a paperback by dimmed lamplight can work wonders, I promise.

NEVER GROW OUT OF NAPTIME

When my twins were babies and toddlers, Kenny and I loved their lunchtime naps. We'd have a quick clean-up after the morning's mayhem and then hop into bed for forty-five minutes of shut-eye ourselves, waking up alert and ready for the afternoon 'shift'. From then onwards I became a fan of the 'mini nap'. I found I could nap for fifteen to twenty minutes anywhere: in the back of a car, on a short train or plane journey, even with the curtains wide open lying on my bed. The risk for some people is that the nap will interfere with their night sleep, so that is why I prefer the 'mini nap'; I think of it as plugging myself back into the mains for a quick top-up as opposed to a full battery charge. If you shut the curtains and snooze for two hours then you may well be disturbing your evening routine and you may wake up feeling groggy and less energetic than you did before.

The Midpointer View

On her episode of the podcast, we found that Claudia Winkleman is a gold-standard napper, even having the odd 6 p.m. nap if she has an evening of work ahead of her. For most people the 6 p.m. nap is, she declared, the 'bungee-jump nap time ... Are you going to come back from it? There's a risk but it's worth it.' Claudia places more emphasis and importance on sleep than just about anyone I have spoken to in over one hundred episodes. I once shared a bed with her at a friend's birthday week-end and because we both had to be up for work the next day, she made us leave the party at 11 p.m. before anyone else, wear eye masks, and then basically told me to shut up when I started waffling on at 11.30 p.m. Her discipline – and love for naps – was inspiring.

'I'll nap in the back of a car. Happily, I'll nap on a train. I rehearse Strictly and then go upstairs and have a nap. A hundred years ago when I was little, my mum happened to sit next to a brain surgeon, and his parting shot to her was, "Do you have kids? Always let them sleep. Encourage them to nap; that's when the body mends itself." So, I had the only mother in the world who didn't say, "Come on, you're wasting the day!" I'm very proud of my naps. I don't understand when we all decided that busy was good. I think busy is not good. And if you allow yourself the nap, don't feel guilty.'

GOOD DAY, SUNSHINE

Spending time outdoors in the morning is also a big factor in a good sleep cycle. Light is really important for our internal clock – as we know with the negative effect of the blue light – so the natural light we are exposed to during the day can help our body regulate what time we go to bed. The first hour of the day is the most important, so even standing with a cup of tea at the back door for ten minutes will help you get that sunlight. We often read about the hours before bed, spraying sleep spray, having warm lavender baths or avoiding caffeine too late in the day, for example, as being very important for our night-time sleep, but our morning routine could be just as important to that sleep success fifteen hours later. In the UK, your time outside won't always be spent in sunlight, but getting vitamin D is very important. The NHS website highlights its links to healthy teeth, bones and muscles, and quality sleep, so consider a supplement if you feel you don't get enough (many GPs now prescribe it for the over-sixty-fives because it's considered so important to good health). Over 20 per cent of people in the UK are vitamin D deficient so you are not alone.

If you start the day pressing snooze four times and then rushing out the door, you have already given yourself unnecessary stress and an excess of cortisol, you probably haven't had the best break- fast and you are unlikely to have exercised or spent time outside. These actions at 7 a.m. are affecting everything that happens at 11 p.m. I know it's boring to bang on about it but it is that word routine again; it's vital.

SET YOURSELF UP FOR SLEEP

I asked sleep expert Dr Sarah Gilchrist for tips on how we can all achieve the perfect night's rest. 'My background is high performance sport. I was a physiologist for Sport Wales and the English Institute of Sport, and a senior physiologist with British Rowing, from Beijing through to the Rio Olympics,' Sarah explained, 'and during that time, I recognised that sleep wasn't really on the agenda in terms of focusing on it for athletic performance. We talked about it, but only at surface level. The English Institute of Sport funded a doctorate, which I completed on sleep and athletic performance, and now I've taken sleep and performance into the health sphere.'

What do you think is the biggest barrier or the biggest problem for people who can't sleep?

'It depends on your age, but certainly understanding that having a strategy for good sleep health is important. So, if I said to you, have you got a strategy to get to sleep? Some people might consider it. I know certainly athletes would've done, particularly athletes I'd worked with because I talk to them about it, but most people in the general population will go, "Well, no, I just go to bed. And if I sleep, I sleep, if I don't ... " They don't consider it. I think of it as the not-so-secret secret weapon. We know we feel better if we sleep, we feel good if we sleep well, but the secret weapon to it is addressing it and having a regular routine and having structure and prioritising it, protecting and valuing it. Our bodies love routine, we're physiological beings. That's how our bodies function. Having a regular get-to-bed time and a regular get-up time is key to getting the right amount of sleep, which is usually seven to nine hours for a healthy individual. And the only way to really assess that is to ask yourself a question: if you wake up with your alarm, do you feel a bit groggy but alert and fully productive during the working day? If not, chances are you probably need to address that sleep strategy a little bit more.'

What advice would you give a shift worker, or a night owl married to a morning lark?

'Communication is key. Sleep is totally individualised. Whether you're an owl or a lark, most people are somewhere in-between, but there are extremes; and then how you react to your sleep, how you react to poor sleep, it's entirely individualised and will change throughout your life. It's particularly difficult if you live with a shift worker as well, because everybody's timetables are completely upside down. If you are in that situation, you've got to talk about it because sleep is the priority. If you're a shift worker, it becomes a lifestyle. Say what you need to prioritise sleep in the day. Put notices on the door to stop the postman knocking, buy blackout blinds, wear an eye mask, keep the phone out of the bedroom.'

And sleeping while those dreaded hormones circulate . . .

'When going through the hormone transitions, the key is recognising what's waking you up. It's entirely normal to wake up and go to the loo a couple of times a night, but obviously during perimenopause or menopause, some of the aspects that you're going to experience, whether it's hot flushes, night sweats, anxiety, depression, can be helped with some practical solutions or gentle psychological techniques; for example cognitive behavioural therapy for insomnia has had some proven positive results. There are lots of relaxation techniques, gentle psychological techniques, practical solutions you could try. What works for one person may not work for another so you need to find what works for you. One example is cooling your body temperature. Body temperature has a circadian rhythm, an internal rhythm like our rhythm for sleep and wakefulness, and we need our temperature to be cool to sleep. So, a cool, calm, dimly lit environment to sleep in will help in getting to sleep or getting back to sleep; for example, a cool room (18–20°C), the right pyjamas, good cotton bedsheets, spare bedsheets. If you wake up, don't put all the lights on and get yourself into a stressful situation, take yourself out of bed and do what you need to do to restore a calm, relaxed and cool state. If hot flushes are disturbing your sleep, things like a chilled pillow are useful.'

The Midpointer View

Mariella Frostrup goes for a soak to sleep well. 'I was always amazed at my husband's mum, who has a bath every night before she goes to bed. I used to think, God, yeah, it's nice to be retired, isn't it? And now I've realised that the nights that I do, I sleep better. We're running around, we're trying to do work, we're trying to run families, we're trying to run the world, and we never, ever take time out for ourselves. If you get into a routine, even if it is just having a bath for a few minutes before you go to bed, even if it feels like it's too late and you've got to be up at six, just taking that twenty minutes out to yourself, sitting there alone in the bathroom with the door locked and your own thoughts is massively important. People will tell you to "do meditation" but a nice warm bath before you go to bed is a form of meditation.'

WHEN YOU REALLY CAN'T SWITCH OFF . . .

I had a very brief period of insomnia in my early twenties, when I started working in radio and I was doing an early-morning breakfast show. I was having to get up at four o'clock, and I couldn't get to sleep because I was paranoid about oversleeping. It got worse and worse, even over a small period of time, and it destroyed me. I can't imagine how it felt for Miranda Levy, author of *The Insomnia Diaries: How I Learned to Sleep Again*, who suffered from a lack of sleep for eight years.

'I'd had a few brief periods [of insomnia] in my life, mainly related to anxiety about a job interview or staying in a new hotel, but this was triggered by an event in my personal life, the end of my marriage, and it then went on to take on a life of its own for various reasons. I was awake for about eight and a half years. It affects you physically. I lost my job, I lost friendships, I temporarily had issues with my family, my kids. I didn't leave the house. I became agoraphobic. But there was another issue, which is important to mention, that I was put on sleeping pills and tranquilisers quite early on and they messed everything up much further.'

I wanted to know how Miranda reclaimed her life – and sleep – after such trauma. How can you get yourself to the stage where you can once again have a good night's sleep? This was her response:

- First of all, I came off Valium. A good doctor won't prescribe you them for more than a week, but too many reach for their prescription pad too quickly because they don't have the time. I had a couple of years of something called post-acute withdrawal syndrome, which is a real thing.
- I got a weighted blanket, which feels like being tucked in as a child, when you were tucked in really tightly so you couldn't move. They are used for children with ADHD and autism.
- I had cognitive behavioural therapy for insomnia. I learnt that you only go to bed to sleep or have sex; you don't do other things. You don't turn your bedroom into a battleground.
- I stopped catastrophising my sleep. I'd think, I'm a good sleeper, but I'm having a bad night. It's not panicking. It's saying, Okay, this is a crap night, but hopefully tomorrow will be better.
- I make a list of everything I have to do the next day, and

I colour code it and I update my list several times during the day. And I do one before I go to bed so I don't need to think about things.

- Exercise is fantastic. In the morning when it's sunny, it affects your circadian rhythm and melatonin levels. Melatonin is a sleep hormone the body produces in response to darkness, and getting outside blocks its production and wakes you up. If you move around more, you're in a better mood, then you get more tired at night. So, get out early, even if it's just for a walk.

As Miranda's story shows us, sleep is very personal and very important. When my kids were little and we were governed by their wake-ups for feeds, and then later by school, I fantasised about a time when we could go back to being night owls. But as they have flown the nest and I am free to control my own patterns of sleep I have realised I am much happier and healthier as someone who gets up quite early and shuts down just after 10.30 p.m. Of course, there's the odd night of letting loose and staying up late, but it's back to that nutritional metric again. Maybe even for sleep it's a 90/10 thing: if we can stick to the routine 90 per cent of the time, we'll probably have enough sleep in the bank for a good, healthy, fog-free life.

Please take sleep seriously. Too often, we think of it as a chore, or something so natural we don't need to consider it. But at our age, often we have to plan to get the best rest. Give yourself the best chance by investing in good bedding and pillows, thinking about what you sleep – or don't sleep – in, and about what you consume (through your eyeballs or mouth) in the ninety minutes before bedtime. Kenny and I believe two duvets are the secret to a long, healthy marriage. Have one each so you don't have to fight, and one of you will never wake up freezing cold because the winner got the duvet in the middle of the night. Other friends swear by getting duvets with different tog levels, and mattresses with different firmness on each side. There's no shame in separate beds or separate rooms. No one longs to be cooped up with a snorer. And rather than being unromantic, it could be sexier, having your own space the other one has to visit.

MIDPOINT ACTION POINTS

- Naps are natural, and totally fine. Allow yourself a few minutes if you feel you need them, and just check in with how it's made you feel at your usual bedtime. Does it hinder you getting off to sleep or are you fine? Listen to your body.
- Educate yourself on the tools out there to help you settle down for the night. Mariella's hot baths and Miranda's weighted blankets are great; you can also try sipping a cup of chamomile tea or a mug of golden milk (warm milk laced with nutmeg, ginger, cinnamon and turmeric) before bed; listen to a soothing book or meditation app; and invest in blackout curtains. Lavender is a restful scent if your senses are craving a pillow spray or bath oil.
- Give yourself the best chance of a good night's rest by taking the experts' advice on calming your mind from this chapter that you know would work for you. If your mind is racing because of worries about work or the kids, make a to-do list before you turn off the light. If mess leaves you anxious, stack the dishwasher and turn it on before hitting the sack. Know what you need, and implement it asap.

8 ILLNESS

The greatest wealth is health.

VIRGIL

Sometime in 2020 when I was forty-seven years old, we heard about the parent of someone at my children's school who had been diagnosed with a rare form of cancer. The friend who'd told us the news paused and said, 'Well, it's Sniper Alley for us now.'

'Sorry?' I said.

'Our fifties are Sniper Alley. If you can get to sixty and manage to dodge the health bullets then you'll probably live well into your eighties or nineties.'

The phrase kept ringing in my ears as, in the couple of years that followed, the theory seemed to be coming true. All around us too many of our peers were dying or being given horrible diagnoses of terminal illness in their fifties. I was already on the voyage of midlife discovery and knew that I shouldn't be eating processed food or drinking too much alcohol (if any at all) and I was happy to keep up the exercise intensity, the three pillars of health (along with not smoking), which seemed to be linked to avoiding disease. Kenny and I felt well. We didn't take our health for granted, and so we added in things like cold water therapy (freezing cold showers for him and some cold water swimming for me) and tried to do breathing exercises occasionally. Health, we knew, was true wealth.

Then, in 2021, Kenny came home from a walk with the dogs having listened to an episode of *The Midpoint* in which I had Davina McCall on as a guest. He walked into my office and said, 'I have just been listening to you and Davina talk about libido and hormones.'

'Yes!' I said, in a way that said, Hurry up. What's your point, caller? I am a bit busy.

'Well, if your libido is helped by HRT, what happens to my testosterone and my libido? Will I be left behind! What happens to men?'

'Men see their hormones drop off at a much slower rate normally,' I answered, hoping that would see him off so I could get back to work.

He looked unconvinced.

'Why don't you get yourself booked in for a well-man check? Get your bloods done to make sure you're happy with your testosterone,' I suggested.

And Kenny, unlike many blokes who might have moved on from these thoughts and onto the next task, booked the appointment – even though he had no symptoms that might lead him to believe his hormones were changing. Kenny has always been the kind to ask about the new product I am using on my face and when we lived in London had regular facials. He is quite keen that I don't steal a march on him in the ageing process, so the fact that he wanted to know as much about his body as I knew about mine and then act upon it was not unusual.

A couple of weeks later he got his results back.

'My testosterone is fine,' he told me. 'But they have suggested I go and see a specialist as my PSA number is a bit high.'

'What is a PSA number?' I asked.

'It's to do with the prostate.'

I don't think in that first conversation either of us thought anything sinister was going on at all. We certainly did not entertain the fact that a year of monitoring and two biopsies later it would be confirmed he had prostate cancer and that in June 2022, at the age of fifty, he'd be having a radical prostatectomy in Guy's Hospital in London.

Prostate cancer is the most common cancer in men. In the UK, 144 men are diagnosed with it a day, and every forty-five minutes one man dies with prostate cancer. It most commonly affects men over fifty and is generally a secondary cancer. Kenny was incredibly lucky to find his cancer early as he had no symptoms, no trouble peeing, no blood in the urine or semen, no problems emptying the bladder, all of which are signs of prostate cancer, but can also be signs of other diseases.

His decision to remove the prostate was made on the basis that at the age of fifty there was a chance the cancer would come back even after successful brachytherapy (a form of radiation) so if he had the prostate removed, he wouldn't be able to get cancer there again, as long as it hadn't already spread. The downside was that the prostate is responsible for releasing the fluid that supports semen and as a result is very close to the nerves that control erectile function. The biggest risk was he'd lose all functionality, and even in the best-case scenario there would be work to do to get himself back fully functioning. He was not going to wake up the day after his operation and be able to get an erection. Because of various physiological measurements and indicators, his consultant said he was confident that Kenny would get something back, but he couldn't say for sure. So, we entered the operation with risk. I say 'we' because when you have been married for twenty-two years, as we had then, and didn't intend to *not* be married, the outcome of this operation was going to affect both of us.

The Midpointer View

Kenny shared how recovery was going on the podcast two months post-surgery, mainly to encourage midlife men to get tested and take their health into their own hands. 'Every week's got better. There're little things that make me feel a bit odd, when you're lifting something or turning around, you accidentally wee yourself. I did start wearing pads because I was paranoid. The first few weeks of recovery were demanding because I'm so used to picking up and doing stuff; I've had many injuries in my rugby career but nothing that stopped me like this. It really did. I struggled to get up to walk. I was sleeping all day, sleeping all night – a little bit snappy with the kids. I think the key thing is to be positive. It could be three to six months before you have normal erectile function but there's a penis pump you can use for ten minutes every day and normal function has returned. Hopefully, my story will encourage you – or someone you love – to get tested. It's not embarrassing to get a blood and urine test, and that's the first step. The finger-up-the-bum test does come later, but the first tests are simple. Talk to your mates. Definitely talk to your mates. Be open. Don't be scared to say how you feel.'

Today, we are eighteen months on from the operation and I am delighted to say Kenny is well and fully functioning, which my kids hate me saying. But it probably took a good eight to ten months to really get his mojo back, and a year before he could say that he was through the trauma of diagnosis and operation psychologically. We recorded a podcast together about our experiences because Kenny said he was so grateful that he listened to the Davina episode of *The Midpoint* that day and he wanted to pay his good fortune forward. If just one person listening to us recommended it to a man they loved, or heard it themselves and felt motivated to get checked out, it might help one person survive and thrive.

PRACTICAL PROSTATE ADVICE

Declan Cahill was the urologist and expert on prostate cancer that Kenny saw while he was ill, and I got him on the podcast for the medical advice men need to keep their prostate in check. 'If you look around most countries in the world, the average life expectancy would be about fifty years of age,' Declan shared. 'We are like the white appliances in the kitchen. We weren't meant to be going far past fifty, and our bladders weren't planned for our prostate to grow and that's why we get some symptoms. Prostate cancer doesn't have symptoms until it's very advanced. The rule of thumb is that symptomatic prostate cancer is incurable, curable prostate cancer has no symptoms. When men go to the doctor because they've got urinary symptoms of poor flow, incomplete emptying, difficulty starting frequency, urgency getting up at night, that's generally due to benign obstructive features of the prostate and that's a common thing for men fifty years plus. It's a fault in a lot of the advertising campaigns about prostate cancer screenings that men with certain symptoms should present to the doctor, because those symptoms are almost never cancer. They're likely of a benign nature. When it's all confined without any symptoms, that's when it's at its curable stage.'

What are your options?

'If you find out you have prostate cancer the options are between watching it – which we did with Kenny initially because we only found some very low-grade tumour, which grows extremely slowly and it doesn't seem to have the power to spread – or take action, carefully considering the consequences of any treatments,' Declan explained. 'With Kenny, he was in the position where we thought he was a fit, healthy individual, he's got a medium life expectancy of thirty years, he doesn't smoke. We could fairly well predict him to be in the 50 per cent of men that make it beyond eighty rather than the 50 per cent that don't. And so, we were thinking that some sort of early treatment would be worthwhile because that would cure him. The problem with that confidence in cure is the more confidence you have in cure, the more risk you have in causing negative impacts. The prostate is an accessory sexual organ, which means it's important for fertility – it produces 98 per cent of the volume of men's ejaculate; and the neurovascular bundles around a gentleman's waterworks are important to avoiding leaking urine when coughing and sneezing, and for the ability to achieve an erection for penetrative intimacy. You've got to make choices between the risk of impact on you and the efficacy of the treatment and the different possible long-term side effects of the treatments, surgery or radiotherapy, or other forms of energy for just treating an abnormal area within a prostate. The holy grail is when the cancer is truly confined to the prostate and you remove it. Because Kenny was young and the cancer was contained, we leaned towards removal because one, we thought we had the expertise to do it and two, he had the well-being to recover well from it.'

Another reason to look after your health, folks: you're more likely to handle an operation and recover from it without complications.

LIVING IN SNIPER'S ALLEY

I didn't see us as a 'cancer' couple. Who does? It's never going to happen to you until it does. Prostate cancer is not a lifestyle cancer; there was nothing Kenny could have done differently to avoid it. But he has now upped his game with more exercise and paying greater attention to what he eats. We had our brush with the Big C and now we are navigating Sniper Alley with even more care and appreciation.

As well as cancer, the big diseases that start to take hold in the fifties are often those that come through longer-term health damage, such as cardiac disease, high blood pressure and arthritis. Some of these are because of lifestyle choices made earlier on in our lives, such as smoking and drinking to excess or eating a high-fat diet, and it goes without saying that the sooner you can eliminate these bad habits the better. It's never too late to improve your midlife health forecast.

In 2021, the Centre for Longitudinal Studies shared the results of a study from the *BMC Health Journal* which showed some worrying trends for those of us born in the 1970s. Among other things, the study found that one in three middle-aged British people had multiple health conditions such as chronic back pain, high blood pressure and mental health issues. The data and research led the author, Dr Dawid Gondek, to conclude that, 'Compared to previous generations the health of British adults in midlife is on the decline.' Studies showed a link between poor midlife health and lower life satisfaction, lower earnings and early retirement, plus a higher risk of having long-term health conditions if you grew up poor. He also said that 'public health guidance should focus on helping the population improve health in midlife so that they can age better, stay economically active and lead fulfilling lives'. As a society we should all be concerned: not only are sick people unable to work and contribute to the economy but they cost the economy more.

The Midpointer View

Jo Whiley is taking her future health seriously. 'I swim for my head and I swim for my body. I do feel at a bit of a loss as to how to look after myself because I'm stiff all the time, but swimming definitely makes me feel a lot looser. I've always thought about yoga, Oh my God, it's just slow, but now, as I'm seizing up and hurting a lot more as I'm older, I'm trying to do a bit more yoga because I know I need it to be more supple. I've got osteoarthritis, so I'm increasingly in pain. I'll be lying in bed at about four o'clock in the morning and all I can think about is my aching bones and joints, and how much agony I'm in a lot of the time.'

THE WORST WORD YOU CAN HEAR

I asked Dr Amir Khan on the show to talk midlife cancers more generally, and what we can do to give ourselves the best chance of not getting them, or recovering if we do. 'The vast majority of cancers are more prevalent as we get older,' he said, confirming what I feared. So, what should we look out for? 'We can look top to toe – this is the way I like to do it, working our way down each system [in the body].'

- In the mouth: if you've had trouble swallowing, any pain, or sticking food as you swallow for three weeks or more, you must go and see your doctor.
- In the stomach: if you're over fifty-five years old and you've got new symptoms of indigestion or heartburn, you must go and see your doctor because both of those require a camera down to look at your food pipe, your oesophagus and your stomach.
- In the lungs: if you've had a cough for three weeks or more, particularly if you're a smoker, but not *only* if you're a smoker, or you're coughing up blood or if you've got any unexplained shortness of breath for three weeks or more, or if you're a smoker with any unusual shoulder pain (e.g. in the back of your shoulder you've got pain

you can't quite explain, you haven't lifted anything funny, and you can move your arm around as you normally would), please do go and see your GP because we need to refer you for a chest X-ray.

- With any unexplained weight loss, we have to think about things like pancreatic cancer. If you're over fifty with a change in your bowel habits, loose motions or constipation, please do come and see us.
- Women over forty, if you've got new symptoms of bloatedness around your tummy, abdominal pain, weight loss, back pain with weight loss, anything that might make you think Have I got irritable bowel syndrome?, that could be ovarian cancer, or another cancer, so please do come and see us.
- Any new vaginal discharge in a postmenopausal woman, whether it's blood stained or not, is unusual and needs to be looked at. We'll rule out infections and thrush first of all, but it could be something like a cancer of the lining of the womb, endometrial cancer, so lots to look out for.

'The list is endless, and weight loss is always a big sign that something isn't right,' he advises. 'That's why if you're worried, come and see us and we will help. What we know about certain cancers, not all, is that there are family links to them. If you've got someone in your family under the age of sixty with cancers, that increases your risk of developing a cancer.'

What can we do to reduce our chances of getting a midlife cancer?

'A number of particular cancers are linked to lifestyle,' he reminds us. 'We have to focus on what we have control of, and some people have more control over their lifestyle than others. How can we reduce our risk of cancer as a nation? How can the government help? Less air pollution, better education, free school meals, bringing nature and exercise into inner-city areas – where air pollution is denser, we see increases in risk of certain types of cancer; we know air pollution can increase risk of lymphoma, in particular – so I'm a big fan of green spaces in inner-city areas. All that fresh air and better food will reduce the risk of developing cancer. I know weight is a sensitive issue for lots of people but being overweight does increase your risk of lots of different cancers, as does processed food, which increases our risk of developing bowel cancer.'

Really, he's telling us what we already know: eat less, and eat better. Get exercise and fresh air. And it's not too late to make these lifestyle changes today.

The Midpointer View

It would seem television presenter Julia Bradbury's midlife has been in many ways shaped by her experience of cancer. 'It doesn't define me, but it certainly was an interesting way to hit midlife: a breast cancer diagnosis. Those are the words that nobody wants to hear. It's a complete shock. It turns your world upside down and there's so much that you have to deal with. But I made a promise to myself once I was through my treatment that I would change things and change myself and certainly look at my health in a different way.'

Julia found renewed mental and physical health through her devotion to getting outside into nature and walking, which is the subject of her latest book. 'The idea for my book, *Walk Yourself Happy*, was in existence before my breast cancer diagnosis because as you've said, I'm quite well known for walking on the Telebox and stuff, and I particularly like walking as a tool for health because I think it is accessible to most people. If you tell people they've got to start weight training three times a week, which I do talk about in the book as well, and you tell them certain things that perhaps would be better for them to eat, it can be very overwhelming. And for a lot of people, I think it's the stumbling block that will stop them getting started walking. I call it a sort of gateway drug to exercise because you can literally start with one foot in front of another. What I've got throughout the book is stories of people who started walking and spending time in nature and it's changed their lives. It's given them an incredible health prognosis and outcome. There's a man in the book who just dug a pond in his garden. He was riddled with arthritis, he was inflamed, he was sore, he was depressed and overweight, so he embarked on this project in nature to build a natural pond at the bottom of his garden, and he learnt other things along the way, including meditation, and he completely transformed his life and his health by doing something like that.'

THE OPPOSITE OF ILLNESS . . .

Sports science and exercise expert Dr Julia Jones' third book is on the topic of longevity. *F-Bomb: Longevity Made Easy* is a study of smart wellness, and simple ways we can boost our chances of living longer and better. 'I've become obsessed with longevity, starting when I was hurtling towards my own fiftieth birthday,' Julia shared, 'and I had come through decades of sport and exercise science, telling everyone to join gyms, and I became fascinated by the fact that fifty years of diet and fitness trends hadn't produced any healthy nations. As the diet and fitness industry revenues were going up, average waistline size was going up, and all the data was just getting worse and worse. I started digging back into research and went on a fascinating journey doing an experiment on myself.'

What did that involve?

'I cancelled my gym membership and I stopped calorie counting, I spent the money on getting a biological age test, getting a gut test and buying a new sleep tracker so that I can start basically gathering data about what was going on in my underlying biology. Thirty years ago, when I was a sport and exercise scientist, I visited the US Navy in California and they showed me how they were using music as a bio hack to reduce anxiety, to boost exercise, endurance, and all of that.' Julia started looking at other bio hacks that could make you healthier, outside of the normal eat well and exercise regime that had dictated the wellness landscape for the previous fifty years.

'If you've got really poor gut health and your sleep quality is terrible, and you've got cortisol constantly coursing through your bloodstream because you're stressed, if you want to go and do a 10k run and improve your time, brilliant . . . But that's not going to offset all the damage that is happening from all these other daily habits that dictate how long you're going to live healthily. We know more about how our phones work than how our bodies work. By learning a little bit about your biology, you can understand why that gym habit is actually negatively affecting your well-being.'

Julia's hacks for a long life

- Diversity in diet is key. We've got this zoo of bacteria in the gut and we need lots of different types of bacteria. The way we eat, with processed foods and repeat shopping, buying the same old things over and over, choosing the same recipes over and over – that doesn't boost diversity. The new guidelines are that we need to be eating at least thirty different types of plants every week to maintain a high diversity of bacteria in the gut, and that is linked to our immune system, that's linked to our metabolism. The gut–brain axis means that the gut microbiome is also driving mental health and cognitive function and inflammation, which is basically your biological age. Try having some kind of probiotic food (like yogurt, kombucha or pickles) and prebiotic food (like garlic, onions and oats) every day because those are the things that the bacteria feed on; otherwise, you're putting live bacteria in and they're just going to die.

- Cold showers give you an excellent opportunity to practise your breath work, if nothing else. Extend the exhales to try to stop the sympathetic nervous system from engaging when you have that sudden change in temperature. And so, to keep control of that, to help train that autonomic nervous system, to maintain a parasympathetic tone, to try to reduce stress chemicals, it's better in the morning and in the daytime. There are some really interesting studies that have shown how people have far fewer illnesses and colds if they are doing cold water exposure – it might be sea swimming, it might be showers.

- The power of music as a bio hack, because the ears lead to the brain, every sound is having an impact on the autonomic nervous system – the brain is deciding whether we're in danger or not. Music is a really easy way to tell the brain that you are safe, to slow breathing down, to slow brain waves down. We've positioned music as entertainment, but listening to music can really help boost sleep quality and act as a metronome when you're doing breath work.

The Midpointer View

Having a stroke changed Olympic sprinter Michael Johnson's outlook on life and death, and his attitude to work and stress. 'I was fifty-one years old when I had my stroke. I don't appreciate life any more than I did before. I've always appreciated everything. Prior to the stroke, when I'm doing my annual medical check-ups and things like that, there's the questionnaire, 'Do you experience stress in your life?' I always said no. I think people experienced a lot more mental issues as a result of stress, but that's not to say that my body wasn't taking it on in a very difficult way and having to deal with all of the stress that I'm putting on it. And that probably contributed to me having the stroke. If we're sitting in a meeting in our conference room at my company's headquarters, and something needs to be done [before the stroke] I'm the first one raising my hands saying, "I'll take that." Well, now I sit on my hands and just look around and go, "Who else?"'

I thought I'd end this chapter by making an exception with someone who is actually a bit beyond The Midpoint but who glows with longevity and good health. Richard Madeley has been a national treasure on our television screens for ... well, quite a few decades now. Yet, he remains the picture of wellness. To end this section on illness with some straightforward and sound advice, I asked him about his secret to eternal youth, and what he's doing in the hope he's got many more years in him.

'I haven't had any serious illness and that's what starts to drag people down, isn't it?' he told me. 'Age-related problems, which you don't get in your thirties or forties, maybe even in your early fifties, but which do start to knock at the door as you move through your sixties and towards your seventies. I'm still basically as fit and healthy as I was when I was forty. They will come and get me in the end, but currently I'm okay, so that's luck, and having good genes. My mother, who died several years ago, when she was in her mid-eighties, looked, sounded and behaved twenty years younger all her life.'

Richard talked about how his dad dying young had changed the way he decided to look after his body. 'He carried too much weight and was a smoker most of his life, and he had a heart attack and died when he was forty-nine. The post-mortem showed his arteries had furred up and he wasn't fit. I vowed then, at twenty-one, I was going to watch my weight. And from that point on, I did. I make sure my cholesterol stays low. I consciously keep my weight down by not eating too much. I don't pig out and I watch how much sugar I have, and I try to watch how much alcohol I drink – but that's my downfall. I drink too much alcohol, and that's now absolutely embedded and ingrained in my day-to-day life. I do push-ups and squats. I don't jog and I don't go to the gym, but I do walk a lot and I keep my aerobic fitness up. So far so good. Low blood pressure, low cholesterol. I get good ECG results every year. You can control those aspects of your life.'

But the smoking . . . ?

'I didn't stop smoking until I hit forty. And then I finally stopped because Judy and I interviewed John Diamond, Nigella Lawson's first husband. He had mouth, tongue and throat cancer because he smoked; it was directly smoking related. We had him on *This Morning* with about three months left to go, and he'd lost about half of his tongue and the top part of the oesophagus, and he was in a bad way. I remember saying to him, "John, you've been very straight about this. Is it because, because you were a smoker?" And he actually said, "Of course, it fucking is!" And I remember

I was going through one of my periods of secret smoking, and I remember at the end of that interview thanking my lucky stars that I hadn't yet suffered what he was suffering and I went back to my dressing room and I reached out to my hidey hole above my wardrobe, pulled out my packet of Benson & Hedges, and not for the first time, I crumpled them up and flushed them down the loo. That was it. I was never going to go back to them because I was never going end up like that. I've never had a cigarette since, and now I'm sixty-five. I'm slightly more at risk of developing a cancer, but certainly I'm free of any heart disease, which is what killed my dad. Smoking is absolutely something you can control.'

MIDPOINT ACTION POINTS

- Without good health, we can't be our optimum selves. Help yourself and cover the basics. You know what you have to do: eat better, sleep better, stop smoking, start moving, drink more water and drink less alcohol. Think about setting yourself realistic guidelines you can follow that will boost your immunity and health: seven hours' sleep a night, eating five portions of fresh fruit or veg per day, getting your heart rate up for three workouts a week, and following NHS guidelines of limiting alcohol to no more than 14 units per week for men and women.
- If you feel ill, tired, or just not yourself – get to the doctor. There is no shame or embarrassment in looking after your health, and an early diagnosis can be lifesaving.
- Start adding small habits and easy routines into your daily life. Walks in nature, a ten-minute meditation, a

cup of green tea, a 10.30 p.m. curfew. All these tweaks can act as building blocks into a better, longer life.

- Treat yourself kindly. You can have the most perfect, healthy life in the world, and you will still get sick or ill at times. You're human. Don't fret or stress that you could have done something differently as you are trying to make sense of it all and recover, just use the information you discovered when you are able to start looking towards the future.

9 HORMONES

Hormones are the music of our bodies, and we dance to their rhythm.

DIANE ACKERMAN

Hormones are important at any stage of life but the midlife is when they really come into focus – probably for the first time since puberty. This chapter is not the complete and comprehensive definition of hormones at midlife, but more my experiences, and the advice and anecdotes I heard on the subject as I was recording my podcast.

As you will have realised by now (if you have read this book in chapter order), our changing hormones play a huge role in so many areas of the midlife mind and body experience which, shockingly perhaps, I had absolutely no understanding of as my body shifted from my thirties into my forties. Before I entered this era, I thought of the menopause as little more than the cessation of periods, which in my mind was no bad thing. I was not someone who attached great emotional significance to them and as I hadn't studied any of the sciences beyond GCSE, I really had no understanding of how the hormonal balance would change in my body or the potential symptoms and outcomes that this would bring. I assumed I'd stay healthy, eat well, up the supplements, exercise and ride on through it all without a hot flush to my name, because apparently that was what my mum had done, 'with Bacardi and Cokes, and dark chocolate'.

My health journey had always been a mixed bag: on the one hand I'd had a regular and unspectacular menstrual cycle with very little in the way of PMS since my periods started at the age of fourteen; on the other, I had unexplained infertility diagnosed at the age of thirty and needed IVF to get pregnant at thirty-one years old. Even after the birth of my twin babies I didn't experience a huge change in my cycle, and I didn't use contraception in the hope that having a pregnancy might have triggered something in my body which allowed me to get pregnant naturally. I was told by my obstetrician that this was quite feasible and had happened to his patients, but sadly not for me.

Therefore, I suppose, discovering that a range of physical and mental symptoms I was experiencing around the age of forty-seven were in fact a period of life called perimenopause was quite a revelation and led me on a voyage of discovery and learning which has been life changing – and in my husband's case potentially lifesaving, as you have read in the previous chapter.

NO SHAME IN SHARING

At the beginning of my journey of openly discussing the menopause I said I felt it was a conversation that men needed to be in on. Any man reading this book now, who has found your way to this chapter, I urge you: please keep reading! The women in your life need you to understand, process and help them on this journey. You might be living or working with someone who could really do with an informed man in her corner; and it's good to have an idea of what is going on with each other so we can be helpful and empathetic. Sharing – and listening – is caring. Also, we will be discussing your hormones, too.

Being open about the menopause can still be considered

controversial. Case in point, I was invited on to a daytime TV programme called *Jeremy Vine* to discuss my philosophy of openness surrounding a subject that I and many others felt had been taboo for too long. One of the callers was a woman in her sixties who vehemently disagreed with me, and said she didn't want men knowing what was going on with her body and that men didn't want to know either. She was alluding to the fact that, by some, women were seen as past it after the menopause; that unable to procreate any more they were barren and cruelly labelled as dried up and useless, by both genders, when what men want is full and juicy, youthful women. This must stop. This narrative has gone on for too long, and has likely held women back from seeking advice and help for decades. I even had a little push-back from my own mum, who in her seventies felt that my generation talk about it too much, and should just get on with it, as she had. 'It's not an illness,' she told some of my friends at my fiftieth birthday party. No, but symptoms can be life-changing and there is no shame in getting help or sharing stories.

The Midpointer View

Feeling confused by your own body? You're not alone. Photographer, special police constable and wife of Rod Stewart, Penny Lancaster couldn't work it out for a while either. 'I hadn't had a period for two months and I was waking up with hot sweats. You feel the heat rising from your feet up your body, like you are stepping into a furnace and you get to the point where you think I can't possibly get any hotter – I'll explode! I would sweat sitting still. It's awful. Then three months later I got another period, and I felt different in my body again. I felt different feelings and emotions. And then it stopped again. And it got to one point during lockdown, my anxiety of cooking every day and doing the home-schooling and all of that stuff, I just had a meltdown and I remember I had a plate of chicken pies and I just threw them across the kitchen and they smashed against the wall and I was in floods of tears, screaming. Rod rushed the boys off, then they came back one by one and hugged me and said, "Sorry, Mummy, we understand."'

Let's be clear: I am definitely not saying menopause is an illness any more than puberty is, but we wouldn't expect teenagers to enter that period of life without an understanding of how their bodies were changing, would we? We certainly wouldn't expect our medics to train to be doctors without understanding teen- age bodies and hormones, would we? So why did 41 per cent of medical schools in the UK in 2019 not have even one minute of their curriculum dedicated to the menopausal period, which can last up to ten years and happens to 51 per cent of the population? Why did those rare medical schools who *did* teach it only devote approximately half a day? This lack of education helps to explain why perimenopausal symptoms can often go misdiagnosed or even missed, and perhaps why only 10 per cent of the population in 2020 who could be prescribed hormone replacement therapy (HRT) were actually taking up the medicine that could help their cognitive function, mood, sleep, libido, heart health, bone strength and many other symptoms affecting the quality of life and relationships.

The lack of understanding doesn't just come from an unwill- ingness to talk, or outdated sexism and misogyny, but probably also lies in a study from the early part of the century which linked increased rates of breast cancer to HRT use. However, further studies have given different results, and as the NHS website now states: 'The benefits of HRT usually outweigh the risks; recent evidence says that the risks of serious side effects from HRT are very low.' Still a stigma clings to HRT, something that could literally be a lifesaver for many women. HRT is not a panacea for menopause but it can be part of the solution for a lot of women and should be something they feel they can discuss with their doctor.

The Midpointer View

Jane Fallon has been helped by HRT. 'I don't mind the principle of ageing, but I did get slightly side-swiped by the menopause at the beginning of my fifties. The first couple of years were a bit tough and I didn't quite know how to negotiate my way through it. I was hot – not just sweating, I used to feel faint and I would sweat from places you didn't even know you had sweat glands. It was just ridiculous. Two years of that, and then suddenly the emotional side kicked in, and I felt absolutely horrific. There was no joy in things that I previously had joy with. I felt like I couldn't cope. I can't remember what – something slightly stressful had happened with work – and it completely tipped me over the edge. I couldn't deal with it and I thought, I don't want to be like this. I don't want to be this person crying, shouting and throwing things around. So, at that point, I went on bio identical HRT [a natural hormone therapy], and that's really helped. I didn't understand why I hadn't gone earlier, but it is the stigma.'

MY MENOPAUSE

I wasn't your classic hot flusher, which was the one symptom I had seen and heard about. The symptoms that got me thinking about what was going on with me were:

- I became a bit more anxious
- My memory started failing me regularly
- My libido slowly began dropping off
- My skin became drier
- I found getting to sleep harder

At first, I put all of this down to ageing. Jesus Christ, I thought, the next forty years is going to be a bag of laughs. But around the time I was experiencing the embarrassing and confusing symptom of brain fog that I wrote about in Chapter 1, a penny dropped. I began to suspect the reason I didn't see that many women presenting live TV beyond the age of fifty wasn't because of their appearance, which I had always assumed was the reason, but because they were losing confidence in their mental dexterity.

Judy Finnigan was a TV stalwart, close to national treasure status when she presented *This Morning* with her husband Richard Madeley for over thirteen years, five days a week, then when they moved to *Channel 4*, and hosted a daily chat show for another eight years. So that is twenty-one years of challenging live television, a genre that tests you like no other. She should have been at the peak of her powers. Then quite suddenly Judy seemed to disappear from our screens. It was all the more surprising as Richard carried on solo, on radio at first and then hosting *Good Morning Britain*. Conspiracies in the gossip columns abounded as to why Judy, who many regarded as the more polished presenter of the pair, the backbone of the duo, had taken a professional back seat at a time when her family were all grown up and leaving home, i.e., at a time when it looked as though she could throw herself into work. A few years later, when she'd been off our screens for a while, she said in a candid magazine interview, 'Menopause can be horrible and mine was, it affected my work badly.' At the time I read her comments I felt sad for her – and us viewers – as she is excellent at her job, but I was not perimenopausal back then, and naively thought, Poor Judy, but that won't be me, I'll eat and exercise my way out of it. Because eating well and upping exercise was how I had dealt with any mental or emotional crisis of the past.

HOW I GOT HELP

I was led to find out some answers about my symptoms by *Midpoint* guest and broadcaster Mariella Frostrup, who had just co-written *Cracking the Menopause: While Keeping Yourself Together* with Alice Smellie. As I read the book, and later when I interviewed Mariella in 2020, I recognised the symptoms she had described from her past as things I was experiencing. Maybe I wasn't going mad after all; maybe I could keep working beyond fifty? When we finished recording the episode, I grabbed the number of her doctor, Sara Matthews, and booked myself in for an appointment at her surgery. Sara did a thorough check on my family history regarding breast cancer, strokes and heart disease and insisted I had a mammogram too, and only then did she offer me the option of HRT. As well as potentially alleviating the symptoms I was experiencing, I was also very interested in the long-term possible health benefits in preventing diseases such as osteoporosis, where bones are more susceptible to fractures as oestrogen drops.

Sara told me, while reading my blood test results, 'Jesus, your hormones are on the floor, I can't believe you're not more exhausted.' But that's the thing about perimenopause: often these symptoms creep up and you get used to feeling a little bit rubbish and a little bit knackered. She prescribed gels, Estrogel (oestrogen) and Testogel (testosterone), and a progesterone tablet which I was to take at night. I felt different within days of starting the treatment. My libido came back to its more normal level, my skin improved, my mood balanced itself and the looming feeling of doom disappeared.

It took me a while to come clean and say openly that I was on something, perhaps for similar reasons to the lady who'd later phone in on *Jeremy Vine*. I was a little reticent – despite knowing how important it was not to feel shame around something so completely natural; something that will happen to half of us. My fear was mainly the ageism in my industry. If I was admitting to being in menopause, would I be cast off? Unlike the woman who called into the TV programme, I didn't care about what men thought of me, apart from my husband – and he was totally on board. Why wouldn't he be with the improved libido?

TIME FOR CHANGE

I questioned my reticence to share my experience when I spoke to Carolyn Harris MP for the podcast, in which we discussed why she was bringing the Menopause Bill to parliament, and she changed my mind: I had to speak up because I had a voice and a platform and many other women don't. Carolyn wanted to help women who were not getting menopause support because of the lack of trained experts available in the NHS, to reduce the cost of HRT, and to make sure GP practices across the UK had someone trained to give guidance, support and address concerns so women could continue to be bright, happy, functioning members of society – for themselves, their families and their communities. The menopause truly is not just about women boosting their libido and feeling a bit happier; it's a societal issue. The economy has lost billions of pounds because women aged forty-five to sixty-five are leaving the workplace.

Carolyn was personally invested in this issue, too. 'It happened to me when I wasn't a Member of Parliament. I was actually working in an office. I told myself that I was having a nervous breakdown. I'd lost my son in 1989 in a road accident when he was eight, so I think I put everything down to the fact that maybe I hadn't grieved properly and I hadn't taken antidepressants at that time, so maybe it had come back to hit me with a force. My doctor responded to what I was telling him [by giving] me antidepressants. I had cognitive behavioural therapy. Then in 2015 I got elected, and started talking to other women and listening to their stories.' A light bulb went on. 'You are in the menopause. That's what's wrong with you.' I'm not saying I'm not in grief. Of course, I am. I'll always be grieving. But I was in the menopause because then I started putting together the facts that I was tired, I didn't have any joy, I was aching all over. I couldn't grow my nails, my hair was getting thinner, I couldn't remember the names of my kids, including the cats!'

I'm sure some of you reading her list will have been there and felt the same. It was this late realisation about her own well-being and healthcare that made Carolyn appreciate how awful the lack of education around the menopause was and how women were suffering in ignorance.

'I thought I was too old for HRT at sixty,' she shared on the podcast. 'It was only when I spoke to a doctor and the doctor said, "If you were a diabetic and you needed insulin, do you stop needing insulin when you reach sixty? Or do you always need it?" And I thought, That's right. If I'm lacking these hormones, then I'm not going to just lack them this week or next week. I went on HRT and it's the best thing I ever did.' And her triumph led her to want to help other women in similar situations. 'I've got a job where I can sit down but if I had had a physical job, I wouldn't have been able to survive. There are a lot of women out there who are in manual jobs, or they're working in shops, or they're doing stuff which is strenuous, and they are really struggling. And they're not getting the support in the workplace: some of them are being sacked because it's been suggested that they're not good at their job any more; or their symptoms have not been taken into account, and they (have to) reduce their hours when they can't afford to.'

This is Carolyn's crusade: to help all women cope with the menopause, and to help *everyone* understand it more. 'A lot of doctors are afraid of HRT. A lot of doctors are not capable of diagnosing the menopause. How many women have been diagnosed with fibromyalgia? Early onset dementia? Osteoporosis, depression, anxiety? Think about the money that's being spent on women repeatedly seeing consultants on different issues. If somebody was to say, "Well, A, B, C and D could be the menopause, let's look at that first . . . " You have to talk about money because that is what so many political decisions will come down to. You can't put a cost on women's health. I am determined to get the word vaginal dryness into every conversation, to do whatever I can to make sure that every woman has the opportunity to continue having an exciting and normal life.' Carolyn – thank you, and on behalf of British women across the land, we salute you.

The Midpointer View

Kerry Godliman knows there's still more educating around this subject that needs to be done. 'The menopause can be very, very up and down. I can't believe how variable it can be. Some days I can barely function and then other days I'm fine. There were things in normal day-to-day life that could floor me, and I could be suddenly excessively emotional about what used to be quite manageable. Not knowing quite how the day is going to fall with energy levels, a bit of insomnia, headaches [is difficult] but the HRT helps manage that. The headaches are definitely under control, and the brain fog and lack of drive. My husband and I talk about it relentlessly. My mum didn't do HRT. I think she was smack in the middle of that health scare so she wouldn't have gone near it; but I am still amazed that I might occasionally chat to someone a bit younger and they'll describe some of their life problems and I'll go, "Have you thought that maybe you should get some HRT?" And they're, like, "No, I'm not there yet." And I think, You probably are!'

WHAT EXACTLY IS HRT?

Many of us feel like our lives have been changed – if not saved – by our HRT prescription. But what exactly is it, and how does it help? I got Dr Louise Newson, a leading menopause expert and the founder of the *Balance* menopause app, on the podcast to answer some questions and correct some misconceptions. 'The first thing to say is HRT stands for hormone replacement therapy, and for most of us who start HRT, when we're perimenopausal, it's not replacing anything. It's topping up the missing hormones. You're just reclaiming what you've lost. The most important hormone is oestrogen, but we also produce a lot of testosterone – there's actually more testosterone than oestrogen in our bodies – and the other hormone is progesterone.'

Explain the bad press?

'For the last twenty years or so, women have been told that HRT causes breast cancer, so women have stopped taking it, healthcare professionals have stopped prescribing it, the media have scared us silly about it; but actually there isn't any evidence that taking HRT [gives] a statistically significant increased risk of developing breast cancer. Well, the big study in 2002 that scared everyone away from HRT was an older type of a synthetic progestogen, actually a type that's in the contraceptive pill that no one seems to worry about. But needless to say, they tried to show there was an increased risk of breast cancer, but when the study was analysed properly, there wasn't a statistically significant increase. It might be a small increased risk, but women get breast cancer regardless of taking HRT or not. It's a bit like saying, "Oh Louise, you clean your teeth every morning and now you've got a sore big toe. Cleaning your teeth has caused your sore big toe." It's an association rather than a cause. Now we prescribe body identical HRT, which is available on the NHS, so it's the same structure as the hormones we are missing. And the studies have shown there's no increased risk of breast cancer, certainly for the first five years. A woman has more risk of breast cancer if she drinks a glass of wine a night, or if she doesn't exercise or if she's overweight. And women take HRT, they often feel better, so it's easier to exercise and lose weight. We know that women might have an increased risk because of their family, but taking HRT isn't going to increase that risk further. And that's what's really important.'

Why do these scare stories need to be debunked?

'It's not just about dying; it's about quality of life. I see and speak to thousands of women who have given up their jobs, their partners have left them, who are suicidal ... and they know it's their hormones. We know around 20 per cent of people lose their jobs or give up their work, or change their work [due to menopause]. We did a survey recently of over three and a half thousand women, and we found that nearly half of them actually wanted to take early retirement or give up work early because of their menopause. When I was perimenopausal, I thought my symptoms were because I was working too hard. I was feeling very tired, very irritable, my memory had gone, my sleep was really poor. One of the reasons we developed our free app *Balance* is so women can be prepared and have the knowledge, but also do their symptom check every three months to pick [the menopause or perimenopause] up early. Because there's no doubt about it, I would've given up my job as a doctor if I didn't have hormones feeding my brain. Life's too short. We need to think about it as a global financial disaster actually, because women are not getting their pension, they're not paying into the economy, and they're wasting a lot of money in services.'

How do you know if you need HRT?

'It's about monitoring your symptoms and seeing if there's any change. I hate to tell you but at age fifty your hormones will not be the same as they were twenty years ago. You can't do a blood test, saliva test or a urine test or wherever people are sold because our hormones change all the time. They're a complete waste of time and money. There are so many symptoms, hundreds of different symptoms, because oestrogen affects every single cell in our body, and often, we are tired because of life. I say to women there are many health benefits of taking HRT and the earlier you take it, the better for your future health – for your bones, heart, brain, and so forth. So, let's try it for three months because it's so low risk and see what happens. Within three months [my patients normally say], "Oh my goodness, that's the best I've felt for ages." And then you've answered your question as to which symptoms are related to the hormones or not.'

The Midpointer View

Lorraine Kelly used her platform, and her morning show, to share stories about the menopause and HRT long before it was in the zeitgeist. 'There used to be this misconception that somehow when you got to the menopause, "you're an old bag, shuffle off", which is the most ridiculous thing in the world. There was this sense of shame to it even five, six years ago. I think that was because everybody felt it was a taboo subject, which is crazy. "Just soldier on, on your own." But how many of [us] were having the worst possible time?'

Lorraine had a rough time with her symptoms. 'My husband didn't know what to do with himself. He didn't know what to do with me. The one thing we've always been able to do is talk to one another and he just said, "I saw you disappearing down a black hole and I didn't know what to do." And it was him who said, "For good-ness' sake, you have to get help." Which is why the next day I basically just sat with Dr Hilary Jones, he listened to my symptoms, and said, "You're menopausal, you silly woman." So many doctors, when you present with symp-toms, go, "Ah, okay, that's anxiety and depression. Here's a pill." Of course, if it is that you need help, but if it's been misdiagnosed that's a real worry.' Thank goodness for lovely Dr Hilary. 'I was finding it hard to get out of bed. I was finding it hard to get that enthusiasm for the job. I found it really interesting when I finally got the patch to slap on my bottom, it was miraculous. Within the space of a couple of weeks, I felt so much better. And I thought, Why did I wait so long? Why did I not recognise this? Why did this sneak up on me? I'm supposed to be reasonably well informed, especially on women's health matters for the show. And if it got me by surprise and snuck up on me, it must be like that for the vast majority of women.' And God bless Lorraine, she's been making sure the symp-toms don't sneak up on her viewers ever since.

IF YOU DON'T WANT TO TRY HRT ...

Some of you may still want to avoid HRT for family history or personal reasons. Talk to your GP about what is right for you, and consider alternative therapies to help with symptoms. Some women swear by cognitive behavioural therapy, acupuncture and yoga to alleviate low mood and anxiety; others change their lifestyle – giving up smoking and/or alcohol, losing weight, exercising more, and giving up things that increase hot flushes such as caffeine and spicy foods. There are a series of homeopathic tinctures and herbs that some people swear help them, such as evening primrose oil, St John's Wort and ginseng, but taking these supplements can interfere with the efficacy of other medications so always speak to your doctor before adding anything to your healthcare plan.

A BRIGHTER FUTURE

I asked my doctor, Sara Matthews, the consultant gynaecologist I was introduced to by Mariella, if women should stay on HRT for ever? 'It's a very individual thing,' she told me. 'Some people like to take a holistic approach and I'm very much in favour of a combined approach myself. There's a lot that diet and lifestyle can do in terms of managing menopausal symptoms but the studies are all out there and we can categorically say that there's nothing as effective for menopausal symptoms in the short term as HRT, and in the longer term, there are probably some major benefits in terms of your cardiovascular health, bone health and possibly for a decreased incidence of dementia, Parkinson's, as well, osteoarthritis, diabetes and certain forms of cancer to staying on HRT. It's very much your own choice, and you could manage potential risks of those diseases in many other ways. But the HRT conundrum has been lifted, and I think it'll be unusual for women not to be on

HRT in another ten or twenty years. How I would see it: I have a thyroid problem and I wouldn't not take my thyroxin. And we've got a bit of a design fault with our ovaries, where they're stopping about two-thirds of the way through your life, so you've got to live a third of your life without your hormones when every single tissue in your body has receptors for oestrogen and progesterone.'

So, HRT will help us live longer . . . and stronger?

'We are hopefully going to live for a very long time, and the aim is to live older – and be *well* as we get older. We certainly know that cases of cardiovascular disease, for example, have decreased very significantly in women who take HRT, and the chronic conditions we see crippling women in their sixties, seventies and eighties – diabetes, dementia, cardiovascular disease and fractures – if we've got a very effective way to prevent those would that not be a fantastic thing? If people want to come off HRT that's absolutely fine. Women will live without (HRT) – some people don't like taking medicines and you can deal with things from a lifestyle perspective – but we will increasingly find that women live better on it.'

I'll keep my repeat prescription then, please.

MALE HORMONES

Although it is women who go through the most turbulent hormonal changes in the midlife, men experience fluctuations too that we need to discuss here. Using the term 'male menopause' is probably a bit too much, but decreased levels of testosterone can increase signs of ageing and other symptoms such as:

- Reduced sexual desire and activity and/or erectile dysfunction
- Decreased energy, motivation and confidence

- Reduced muscle bulk and strength
- Height loss
- Sleep disturbances

I had Dr Pixie McKenna as a guest on the podcast to give some advice to men about their hormones and what to watch out for. 'Men's hormones don't jump off a cliff – unfortunately for women, because that's why they don't always understand us when our hormones jump off a cliff,' she said. But male hormones *do* change. Testosterone reduces between approximately 1–2 per cent every year between the ages of thirty to forty onwards. 'It's really a slow burner, but it can have quite dramatic effects. They get some similar things to menopausal women: night sweats, loss of libido, issues with their hair. They can carry weight in places they don't want it; they get the man boobs and the tummy fat. Some men can become anxious or depressed. They feel like they've lost their mojo in terms of their ability to carry out tasks or even remember things.' As she listed the symptoms, it all sounded very similar to what women of the same age group go through during the perimenopause.

How can men find help?

'There are things that can be done if after having a series of blood tests, your testosterone is low.' Pixie's advice is to go and talk to your GP, share your concerns and push for tests. She also urges men not to be ashamed to share symptoms, even stereotypically embarrassing issues such as erectile dysfunction. There can be lifestyle and pharmaceutical help on offer if you ask for it. Get informed. And thankfully for men, getting something to help erectile dysfunction is a lot easier than it has been for women getting HRT. There are some risks to consider (it may increase the risk of heart attack, blood clots and stroke), so talk to a doctor about signs and symptoms and the pros and cons of testosterone treatment.

A BRIGHTER FUTURE

The menopause is a topic that will be important to everyone as they approach midlife: the women experiencing it and the men who are married to or being mothered by – or working with – a woman going through it. We must keep up the good work of breaking down the taboos and increasing understanding. And now we know: men need to watch out for their hormone levels, too.

The day after Carolyn Harris MP's bill had been read in parliament, I was asked to appear on BBC *Breakfast* as a supporter of hers, and by now I was speaking very openly about my own experience. It was a perfectly nice interview discussing what menopause is and how it can deliver over thirty-five different symptoms to women and what we can do to help ourselves.

Later that day my husband was attending an international rugby match at the Principality Stadium in Cardiff.

As he took his seat two men in their sixties next to him nodded a hello.

'We saw your wife on breakfast TV today,' one of them said.

'Oh yes,' Kenny replied.

'She was talking about the menopause. Do you believe in all that?' one of them whispered to him.

Kenny chuckled and then like a true ally told them not only why he believed it, but why it was important that they also knew about it if they had any women in their lives. They seemed converted by his response and happy the menopause was indeed real. I hope they are out there now, spreading the word about the menopause, at their golf clubs, local pubs and on football stands. We all need to be in this together.

MIDPOINT ACTION POINTS

- First of all, hormone changes and fluctuations affect us all, men and women, in different ways; and neither the brain fog that got me, nor the insomnia, weight gain, nor any of the other symptoms that can come as part of the perimenopausal package, nor the lack of libido that gets many men will be universally experienced by everyone. That doesn't mean it's not real.
- Don't feel any shame about changes you feel in your body. If you share your issues, you will find support. For decades now, doctors and scientists have been studying this subject, so that we, today, can honestly feel better about the future and our hormones. Timing is crucial. If you think you might be experiencing symptoms, please go and talk to your GP. Don't live in denial. It won't disappear. Studies show that if you start taking HRT at the right time, you get a much better effect in reducing cardiovascular disease, osteoporosis and dementia, and likewise if you start taking a testosterone supplement at the right time, it may have positive effects on bone density and memory.
- Remember if you're reading this as a younger person, a decade or so before the big hormone drop-offs begin, your diet, lifestyle and any excess weight you carry can have an impact on physical and mental symptoms you may incur, so get ready by being in the best shape you can be as you approach your midpoint.

10 ALCOHOL

Here's to alcohol: the cause of, and solution to, all of life's problems.

HOMER SIMPSON

Let's start with some maths. If you started snaffling a bit of alcohol from the family drinks cabinet around the age of fifteen and you're now fifty years old, you've been drinking alcohol for thirty-five years. Now I appreciate that in the teenage, illegal-drinking years this was in no way a consistent habit and if I am talking about me, which I am, then I was actually not even much of a drinker at university (I probably got tipsy at formal dinners a few times a term if at all) . . . but still, that's a lot of booze over the years.

When I was younger, I didn't have much of a taste for it and was quite happy to be the designated driver. My first job in local radio saw me wake at 4 a.m. every day of the week and my boyfriend was training hard to get into the SBS arm of the Marines, so I didn't drink then either. However, when I moved to London for my second job at the age of twenty-three, the floodgates opened. I was newly single and didn't know anyone when I arrived, so my new social life revolved around after-work pubs and accepting invitations to boozy parties. There were a few fun-filled years of weekend partying and big midweek dinners, because in my twenties I could quite easily stay up until 3 a.m. and then work the next day. You were probably the same.

After the birth of my babies, I'd already dropped most of the midweek parties and boozy weekends but slipped into a few years of enjoying a bit more alcohol at home with my husband. The 'fancy a bottle of wine with dinner?' habit lots of couples have when the babies have gone to bed was very seductive a few nights a week – although we were always mindful that one of us should be under the limit to drive in the case of an emergency, so at least we had that handbrake. Then when the kids got bigger and started eating with us, having homework and going to bed later, the wine at home stopped, or slowed down, and I don't think my drinking habits or patterns will be wildly dissimilar to many people my age with kids and a job. I am definitely not a big binge drinker, but it's always been around.

In my mid-forties I noticed I was not able to process alcohol in the same way. White wine was no longer my friend and the hangover started to appear before I had even gone to sleep. I've since learnt that I was not imagining this: as a midlife woman my body was not producing the quantity of enzymes I needed to break down alcohol at the same rate – and add to that the fact the liver shrinks as we age, which is the organ processing all the alcohol. If it's smaller it is going to take more time to do its job efficiently and I could feel it. Anything more than one large glass of white and I was almost certain to wake up groggy and needing a nap later in the day.

The Midpointer View

News presenter Charlene White no longer wants to deal with hangovers as she settles into midlife. 'I was talking to other mums about this: it's the fear of having one drink too many when you've got young kids because you've got to deal with them in the morning, and there's a one drink difference between it being okay and it being absolutely horrendous to have to deal with them the next morning. So, I will go out for dinner and then it'll get to a point where I'm, like, "I want to go home." I had my friend's fortieth a few weeks ago and we'd gone to this great Chinese restaurant near Baker Street and we'd done a shot. Everyone was in a really good place, and [saying], "Let's go to karaoke in Soho." I said, "I'm just going to get a taxi home because the thought of getting home at three o'clock in the morning and then my kids getting up at half past six, I won't enjoy karaoke. Have a lovely time." I felt amazing when in the group chat [the next day] everyone's, like, "I'm hanging. I feel awful. Why did we do that?" That is why I was sensible.'

FAMILY TIES

My dad has been a problem drinker for a few decades, spending time in rehab and hospital, so I have always been very mindful about alcohol and the effects it has not only on the drinker's health and life, but on those around them. I had seen up close what it looks like when alcohol is in control, and I did not want to go there. As my forties wore on, I started questioning my drinking habits, and when I began to see friends drop it altogether and not only survive but thrive it made me think even more deeply about the societal pressure to drink, and how it was making me feel. I'd do Dry January occasionally to prove to myself I was totally fine without it and when I worked on things like the Olympics or World Cups, I often stayed off it altogether or only had a G & T at the weekend. It's very easy to slip into drinking every day when you work abroad; there is an air of the ex-pat about it all. But my forty-something face was keeping me on the right side of drinking too much. I knew I couldn't go on telly and look my best after a big night any more. Vanity, rather than a desire to protect my organs, drove my altered habits.

I started to see more and more accounts on Instagram and then more apps, books and articles dedicated to helping people stop drinking. This advice was not aimed at people like my dad, but at people who are known as 'middle-lane drinkers' like me. I persuaded some of the experts behind these apps to come on the podcast and was impressed with their enthusiasm and strategies for a sober life. It all made perfect sense.

DRINKING UP GOOD ADVICE

Alcohol is one thing that goes hand in hand with socialising, isn't it? And when many of us find our relationship with alcohol changing in midlife, we worry it will hold us back from going out, dancing on tables, having fun with our friends. So, I spoke to Matt Pink, aka Better Life Guy, about how sobriety can impact relationships. 'I'm three years deep into this journey. Year one was about staying away from everything, reassessing who I was. Year two was about rebuilding and rediscovering who I actually am, because [as] you go through life and you walk into a new school, or a new job, you've got to become a new person; you've got to become like [your new friends]. We build these shells like an onion, and what happens when you stop drinking is you're just left with all these different layers to unpeel to figure out again, Who am I? And that takes a period of time. And now year three, I'm kind of like, "Okay, I've got rid of the booze. I know who I am. I know what I want to do with my life." I'm giving back to people. I don't know what years four, five and six are going to look like, but I'm going to be honest about it the whole way.'

Matt's top tips on maintaining relationships during these years of sobering change

- Those around you might resent it, but do it anyway if it's right for you. 'People are scared because when people think about giving up drink, everybody they know around them drinks.' But have faith in your truth, that stopping boozing will be good for you.
- Prepare yourself for loss. '75 per cent of the people that I drank with disappeared on the spot. That's a fact. But I would say out of those people, half of them three years later have come back and I think it was an initial shock.'
- The good friends will come back to you, in a different way. 'But it's been really nice to welcome those people back. We've met for lunch, for coffee, for breakfast. We've gone for runs.'
- You can help them change. 'Some of [my friends] have ended up giving up drinking, which is why they sort of ran away [from me] in the first place. It's a little bit like holding up a mirror.'

BUT BOOZE IS SO TEMPTING . . .

And yet with all that knowledge as I write this, I am still a 'drinker' in as much as I will, at some point over the next couple of weeks, have a drink or two. Even though I know that the best way to prevent almost every disease and illness would be to cut it out altogether. The NHS guidelines still say fourteen units of alcohol spread over three nights of the week would be classed as 'safe drinking'; that's six medium-size glasses of wine, which I reckon on average I safely adhere to. But there are many other experts and health gurus who suggest there is no safe limit, alcohol is toxic and the body has to work so hard to process it, so why would you add the extra stress on to it?

Nutritionist Rhiannon Lambert explained why Charlene and I had started to feel so bad with alcohol as we got to The Midpoint. 'As we age, our bodies slow down, and because we've got such a slow metabolism as we age – and I know this sounds very depressing but it's the fact of life – unfortunately we do need to start limiting alcohol because it will stay in our system for a lot longer. You could feel the effects [more], and that's because your body's not eliminating it fast enough any more. You've also got depletion of cells and depletion of water, meaning you'll feel more dehydrated.'

For menopausal women who often struggle with sleep it would seem to be a no-brainer to cut down on alcohol, which has a terrible effect on the quality of your sleep and can also increase anxiety the day after a glass or two. And for many men in midlife, it seems cutting back on the beers to lose weight, which is often the prime motivation, can lead to an increase in other healthier habits and a realisation that life is better without it.

The Midpoint View

One of the most evangelical non-drinking guests I have had on the podcast is the comedian Lee Mack, who stopped drinking seven years ago. He is passionate about how our societal narrative on drinking is perverse and is convinced that in thirty years' time we will look back and wonder how we let drinking so much become so culturally normal. 'Someone said, or I read somewhere, that alcohol doesn't get in your bloodstream for twenty minutes. I remembered that feeling, Friday, after work, you take a big gulp, and you go "ahhhhh", as if it was having some magic alcohol effect on your brain. But that's impossible because it's not in your bloodstream yet. So, what is really causing that? There are theories – it's the first time you've sat down all day, it's the first cold drink you've had all day, it's the first time you've stopped working all day, or you're in a nice place with your mates. There are all sorts of psychological reasons you could feel better for that drink – but it definitely isn't the alcohol. The first drink I'd have would be a soft drink, a pint of blackcurrant and ice. I'd drink that, and when you do that for the first twenty minutes, you're not quite as bothered about that [alcoholic] drink as you were, because all the real reasons you were drinking have been done anyway. Giving up [booze] is a phrase used a lot, as if you've sacrificed something, as opposed to gained anything. But the list of [benefits] you get from [stopping drinking alcohol] is so much bigger. You're not giving up as much as gaining! I could probably have a drink now and it wouldn't massively bother me. I don't not drink because I'm trying to battle it, I just think about it differently now.' He doesn't want to drink because he knows that he feels better without it, and that most of us would. My guess is he'll be proved right.

TAKE A BREAK?

Behaviour change coach and founder of the sober life app *Dryy*, Andy Ramage, says it's those of us like Lee, in the middle lane – we're not addicts, but we drink a few glasses regularly, and the alcohol makes us tired, inconsistent, grumpy, and negatively changes the way we eat and sleep – who are the ones who could really feel the benefits quickly of cutting out booze. We've got the biggest gains. He suggests that if we take on the challenge of Dry January or Sober October, and notice how we feel more alert, energetic, and make better choices, we may then decide to make a positive, permanent change in our life, and ban the booze.

There's no doubt when we are conducting our midlife MOT and looking at the ways the reboot might benefit our older selves, then the column marked alcohol should be looked at honestly and carefully. It seems when it comes to booze, it's not about what you're giving up, it's about what you gain.

MIDPOINT ACTION POINTS

- Stopping drinking can feel like a lonely endeavour in our society. Seek out sober life communities, online, or even in the newly springing up bars and restaurants. More people would love to stop drinking, or have secretly given up, than you can even know.
- Don't go all or nothing at first if that feels daunting – set yourself the challenge of a booze-free month, or season, or stop drinking during the week, and notice the changes in how you're thinking, feeling, eating and sleeping. Big positive impacts will persuade you to try more periods of drinking less.
- Alcohol is the only drug that friends and family can frown on you for trying to give up – maybe you're making them question their own choices? Be strong, and know you'll get kickbacks. Be prepared by taking on the role of designated driver (everyone is grateful to those), or adapt your social life so it's not all about sitting in the pub nursing a gin and tonic, but more about going to the theatre or cinema, or doing exercise with friends, activities where alcohol is not socially expected.

PART THREE

What is happening in our lives?

11 STYLE

Don't be into trends. Don't make fashion own you, but you decide what you are, what you want to express by the way you dress and the way to live.

GIANNI VERSACE

I learnt the hard way that style isn't fashion. When I first started out in TV in the late nineties, I worked briefly with a stylist who was in her late forties. I was twenty-three years old, full of youthful sass, and thought I knew what suited me and how to buy clothes. I did not. I had a wardrobe of eclectic nonsense and as I earned more money, I made the mistake of believing that if I paid more for my clothes, then somehow I'd acquire chic-ness. Occasionally, by accident, I bought something which had quality and style, but most of the time I didn't get it right. For my twenty-fourth birthday party I bought a Voyage cardigan (these were outrageously priced items favoured by the boho Primrose Hill set of the nineties, which were made of second-hand materials with ribbon borders and large contrasting buttons); I styled it with a pair of tight denim pedal pushers and a pair of kitten heels. A boy I really fancied declared I looked like Widow Twankey, the pantomime dame, as I walked into my own party. He was right. Hopefully my terrible style is behind me now. Yes, that is a pantomime pun.

Around this period of wandering the style wilderness, I met

the previously mentioned female stylist, who was asked to dress me for a big TV Awards event at the Royal Albert Hall. She had a beautifully cut silver-grey bobbed hairstyle, strong features not unlike Anjelica Huston, and was one of the most put-together women I had ever seen – and it wasn't just me who thought she looked great. I noticed that when we walked down the street, she turned the heads of women and men of all ages. As the daughter of a glamorous midlife woman, of course I wasn't immune to the idea that anyone over the age of twenty-four could be attractive, but what I realised being around this older woman was that style is more than the items we wear; and that what this woman oozed was class, confidence and a strong sense of self. Unfortunately, they didn't sell all of those qualities in Selfridges, so instead she dressed me in a fabulous Jean Paul Gaultier black tuxedo dress. I felt amazing in it that night, and I had learnt a big lesson about style in the process.

The next seminal moment in my style journey was when I started working with Charlotte Green, who is now one of my close friends and my forever stylist. She offered to come to my house and do a clear-out of my wardrobe before we did a 'work' shop together. We packed up sixteen black bin bags of clothes to donate that day. At the end of her cull, before we bagged up the clothes, there were three piles on my bedroom floor. One was called 'Keep', one 'Debate' and one 'Throw Out'. Things didn't start well when she asked me to work out which pile was Keep and I chose the Throw Out. On the Debate pile was a skirt which I had bought in Singapore airport from a designer called Shanghai Tang.

'What is this?' Charlotte said as she held up the offending item, a pale blue chiffon ra-ra skirt with random pictures of a medusa type head on it.

'I've never worn it, actually; but I thought it was something that Kate Moss might wear,' I suggested.

'But *you* are not Kate Moss!' she replied.

Over the twenty years since we have had some interesting edit days but that was the most brutal and hilarious. Charlotte helped me to curate a wardrobe that wasn't full of last-minute panic buys but consisted of excellent basics and a few statement items which, as she put it, 'might cost a lot now, but you'll be handing them down to your [unborn] daughter' – and she was right. Lois, my daughter, wears the clothes and uses the handbags from that period, which gives me great joy. Especially when I work out the £-per-wear rate.

LESSONS IN STYLE

These days I do about two big shops a year and buy very little in-between. What reaching my midpoint has brought me is a greater sense of confidence in the clothes I wear and a better understanding of what suits me.

- While my weight might not be dramatically different to my thirty-year-old self, I know my midlife body is packaged differently. So, it's important to dress the body you have now, not the one you had then.
- The length of skirt I choose is longer, especially if I want to wear bare legs, as no matter how much I train there is a difference in the skin on my thighs and above the knee which I am not overly keen on sharing.
- Having once loved them, I don't wear low-waisted jeans and I don't want things that are unfeasibly tight or restrictive. I want to move as elegantly as possible, not be restricted by my clothes.
- Look at what the 'kids' are wearing but don't try to ape it. Make their trends your own. I think anyone who has a teenage daughter changes their attitude to how they dress because there's this little person on your shoulders all the time, influencing you or being influenced by you.

- I know a well-cut suit is forever and buying new all the time is unnecessary and wasteful. I'd rather wear a dress I have worn three times before and pay to get a blow-dry for a special occasion than buy something new just for new's sake.

These lessons are all hard-learnt and quite a big shift from those early haphazard fashion days of my teens and twenties. In the distant past I was that person who went out for a lunch date in one top, decided she didn't like it on the way there and then bought a new one in a panic and changed in a toilet. Talk about not knowing who you are.

STYLE COUNCIL

Of course, I had to get my super-stylist Charlotte on the podcast and into this book to share her sartorial wisdom with everyone. If she can sort me out, she can help anyone. What does she think about midlife style – and what we can do to stay visible and confident in this tricky era of change? 'I think we get to a certain age and we think there's a new set of rules that we have to follow,' she says. 'And I think we really have to kind of stick to the essence of what we're about. We don't have to suddenly put a shift dress or a wrap-around dress on. We can still be fashionable. Our bodies may change but we can accommodate that, and I think it's very important that we're comfortable in what we're wearing when we go out that front door. The old rules have gone out the window. Denim, for example – you can wear that at any age now. You may wear it in a different way, but I think a white shirt, a jean and whatever shoe, you're going to look stylish, you're going to look cool whatever age you are.' If in doubt, simple basics are always a good place to start.

Charlotte's three universal fashion tips

1. Edit religiously. I think you really need to make
    that wardrobe work for you. An item of clothing is
    allowed to sit in your wardrobe for about a year if it's
    something that might not get an outing often, like
    an expensive evening dress, but with everything else
    every six months I go through and think, Have I worn
    it? Do I need to rework that? Can I rework it? Can I
    try that with something? Sometimes I have a good old
    dressing-up afternoon just to challenge myself to see
    does that go with that? Is that appropriate? You need
    to make that wardrobe work for you because it saves
    time. It's just easier. Everyone has busy lives.

2. Invest wisely. When you've done that big edit, I think
    it's so important to invest. You need to buy now, wear
    for ever. So rather than spend a little amount on a
    bargain jumper, which you might only wear for a few
    months, spend a bit more on something that you'll
    have in your wardrobe for years. Go for something
    quite neutral that you can wear smart or casual. You
    can really make pieces like that go a long, long way.

3. Enjoy your style. Be brave, be confident. The other
    day my daughter and I were going out the door and
    we had the same tracksuit bottoms on, and I had this
    moment of fear of being mutton dressed as lamb . . .
    And then I realised we were wearing it in a totally
    different way. I was wearing flats and a polo neck, and
    she had a rather cropped puffer and a chunky trainer.
    I realised we could both go out in the same tracksuit
    and it was fine. I still felt myself and she felt herself.

MEN'S FASHION

I probably spend more time these days addressing Kenny's wardrobe woes than my own. He thought he'd found the fashion panacea a few winters ago when he bought almost everything on the Reiss website . . . Then realised loads of his friends around the same age as him had done the same thing so they all looked identical when they went out. Considering he doesn't wear suits for work he was also left wondering why he had acquired fourteen white shirts and fourteen pale blue shirts, all of which he'd carefully colour coded in his wardrobe. The kids mock his attempts to get the right trainer, a new pair drops through the door every couple of weeks and still they tell him that they are not quite right. If I say his trousers look nice, he'll buy the same pair in four different shades of beige and always one in navy blue. He's resorted to telling me he wants clothes every birthday and Christmas so I can be responsible for his 'look', and taking on the responsibility of these twice-yearly shopping trips is when reality hit home: it is hard dressing a midlife man, especially one who wants to look good but not like he's spent all day getting ready. They don't dress how their fathers did in midlife, but they don't want to look like they fell asleep in their teenage son's wardrobe either. Comfort is king, but can you really wear a tracksuit all day when you are fifty-one? Well, Nihal Arthanayake said you can when he came on *The Midpoint*, but he's a former rapper and has a confidence with clothes which is rare for a man over fifty.

For a while, I tried to give Kenny focal points, a few clothing heroes, and I'd say to him, 'Think to yourself, Would Daniel Craig wear this?' His response was generally along the lines of, 'I don't care what he's wearing, he's got a stylist, a six-pack and a massive budget.' Fair enough.

Before giving up, I called Sinead McKeefry, who has dressed some of the most well-known men on TV and an array of music stars (as well as being the woman responsible for Claudia Winkleman's iconic *Traitors* wardrobe), and asked her for some midlife men styling advice. Here's what she shared:

- Midlife men should not wear a stiff leather jacket in any shape or colour. Soft leather is okay. If you own a stiff one, give it away.
- Unless you are Iggy Pop, never ever wear a skinny jean.
- Sporty men (think David Beckham) can wear any tracksuit they like, any make, any colour or brand. However, the slightly less sporty man should go for a more understated look. Get inspiration from Cos or Uniqlo.
- Look for brands that do the classics well but also give a nod to seasonal fashion trends. Invest in a good Crombie coat, a great cashmere knit and some well-cut jeans, which will see you through many winters, then you can add the odd fashion item. Cos and Reiss for T-shirts and chinos on the high street.
- When it comes to trainers, stick to sports brands rather than a fashion brand: Nike (Air Max 1 and low Blazers), Vans, Adidas (Samba and Gazelle) and New Balance, who do great colours.
- If you only buy three things let these be them: a navy cashmere round-neck jumper (M&S do these), Levi's 541 cinch-back mid-denim jeans and a pair of brogues.

The Midpointer View

Nihal Arthanayake wants to give men his age a pep talk: if you love it, wear it; who cares what anyone else thinks?

'There's nothing stopping any man in his fifties from dressing how he wants other than the fear of someone else's opinion. But if you don't care about anyone else's opinion in this regard, and I don't, then you're good. It doesn't matter.'

YOU GOT THE LOOK

Midlife is often a time for reinvention and reimagining lots of things about ourselves and our lives, but I don't think middle-aged people should throw what they have learnt about style out of the window just because they hit a landmark birthday. The idea that we need to adopt elastic waistbands and fade into the background is not being entertained round here. Why? Because I truly believe spending time on your appearance and thinking about what you wear and what suits you is not frivolous or an expression of vanity, it's about feeling the best version of yourself, and the outfit you choose can be an added layer of armour for the days when your confidence might not be so strong.

HONESTY IS A HOT TREND

I am a great believer in planning ahead. Perhaps once a week, or month, or at the start of every season, think about taking a couple of hours to go through your drawers and wardrobe and try your clothes on to work out a few outfits for the weeks ahead. What doesn't fit right, what needs to be cleaned or ironed, what is damaged and needs repairing ... It's a good use of time and will help you avoid any early-morning panic dressing or holiday packing. Another key thing is to be honest with yourself about what is not suiting you. Stop telling yourself that when you lose a few kilos, you'll be back in that skirt, or that one day you'll be invited to an event that requires a fluorescent pink plastic catsuit (you won't). Be brave, be truthful and cull. Yes, you may lose a few kilos, but dress for the body you have today, or you'll have a wardrobe full of clothes that don't fit and you'll be subliminally telling yourself that who you are now isn't good enough. You probably have that one mate who always seems to get it right when it comes to clothes, or a discerning daughter or husband. Send them a few pictures and ask for honest feedback. And then, more importantly, notice what makes you feel good.

ALWAYS IN VOGUE

Who better to talk about style at midlife than Alexandra Shulman, CBE, the longest-serving editor in the history of *Vogue* magazine? Alexandra has learnt how to work with her body, confidence and wardrobe as she's got older. 'When I went to *Vogue*, I knew I would be scrutinised, that I would become more of a kind of public figure, and I was kind of okay about that, but I think if I'd been thinner-skinned than I am it would have been quite hurtful,' she confessed on the podcast. 'I got fed up with the way I was portrayed as somebody who wasn't like you'd expect the editor of *Vogue* to be ... and people were still writing that after twenty-five years. Well, hold on a moment. What do you expect? I've been editor of *Vogue* for twenty-five years, so this is what the editor looks like!'

When it comes to style, Alexandra was reminded on a recent holiday that often the key to a great look is owning it with confidence. 'On the beach last week, I'd noticed [with] the bikinis there's a big kind of thong thing going on, so everyone's bottoms are hanging out. I was thinking, Oh my God. Even at seventeen I couldn't have done that! My bottom is not nearly nice enough!

There was a woman, probably in her seventies, possibly even eighties, a large woman, wearing one of these thongs and my first thought was, Ooh, I don't know if that's a good look! And then I immediately went into self-correct. Because actually it's fantastic that she feels so confident with herself and able to potter around. She wasn't trying to be glamorous. She had come down for her daily swim and felt completely happy walking around with her body.' Again, confidence is your sexiest, most stylish fashion accessory.

What are Alexandra's tip for looking good at any age? 'I used to wear low-cut things and I had a figure that suited fifties hourglass clothes. I'm sixty-three now, and don't wear that so much now. This is the bit of getting older that isn't brilliant: your shape is not what it once was. But I think what is important is those little things that make a difference between you looking [stylish or] rather frumpy. It is to do with a heel height that you are wearing, or where the waist or sleeves of a dress falls. I've really noticed paying attention to those kinds of little micro trends is all the difference between looking like you've got stuck in a time warp.'

SHOP TILL YOU DROP

The queen of British shopping is Mary Portas – she has sorted out leagues of British people's style over the last few decades – so I asked her for some general style tips. 'We've become much more relaxed about fashion and how we wear it,' she says. 'I just put on what I like; it's about a feeling. If you feel good, you wear it – that's the only thing I can say to people.'

More golden nuggets of advice from Mary . . .

- The worst thing is trying to follow the trends and thinking, That's what I want to be. Knowing what fits you, what looks good on you and what you feel relaxed in comes from within.

- Simplicity is key. Find about two or three pairs of trousers that you absolutely love; looking at them when you're buying them, going, How will that look with a great trainer?
- Wear things looser as you get older, you don't need too tight. You know, you don't need to work like that. We don't need to, so just keep it loose. It looks sexier.
- If you're tired, put on glasses – that often helps.
- There's also simplicity in great pieces of jewellery.

MIDPOINT ACTION POINTS

- Are you set in your style ways? Now is the time to spice things up. Ask for help – ask a friend whose fashion sense you admire, flick through some fashion mags or follow some stylists you like on Instagram.
- Declutter more than your wardrobe. Go through your jewellery box, your shoe cupboard, your winter coats, and don't keep things you don't utterly love, use or keep saved for sentimental value. Lightness will help you dress in a hurry.
- Don't overthink your look every time you leave the house – remember Mary's rules ... think about what feels comfortable and boosts your confidence and you can't go far wrong. You be you. Everyone else truly *is* taken.

12 LOVE AND SEX

Life is short. Kiss slowly, laugh insanely, love truly and forgive quickly.

PAULO COELHO

Romance is a very subjective topic. One person's romantic dream of having rose petals laid over their bed and sprinkled into the bath is another person's hoovering and plumbing nightmare. From the unscientific observations I've noted over the last half-century, I think being appreciated, heard and seen is often a more powerful indicator of the long-term success of a relationship than enormous romantic gestures. I say half a century because often the first lessons we learn about relationships come from the environment we were brought up in, and what we see our parents, grandparents and siblings doing in the love arena. That doesn't mean your partner has to be the offspring of Eros for them to have a clue about romance, nor does it mean you will repeat the patterns of your parents' relationship if they weren't Cleopatra and Mark Antony, but a lot of the rituals and dynamics you witness at home about love and how to be in a relationship will stick with you. You may want to re-create them, or not, but they will linger in your psyche.

Case in point: my husband Kenny is a romantic man (lucky me) but I think this may be a reaction to the lack of 'gesture' romance he felt there was in his parents' relationship, and his aim to self-correct. As a ten-year-old, he would cycle to the local garage to buy a bunch of flowers for his mum if his dad had forgotten a significant day and then give them to his dad to present to his mum. His dad was a dairy farmer and woke at 4 a.m. every day, so his parents slept in separate rooms, and Kenny has an aversion to us sleeping in different rooms. He'd rather be woken early by me than for us to sleep alone. He's totally fine about me going away for work for weeks on end but at home he's not up for separate beds, and I am sure this goes back to childhood memories of his parents' separate bedrooms, and how that made him feel.

In the first throes of a relationship, the large bunch of roses that arrives *just because* is a beautiful gesture, but if flowers then arrived on repeat on the same day every week thereafter it would eventually lose meaning. It would become just a standing order. The gesture would soon become a chore, expected, lacking in thought. Being appreciated, heard and seen, however, never gets repetitive.

Sometimes, we can get it wrong in the romance stakes – even when we mean well. A friend of mine knew that she needed to have a chat with her husband when he bought her a Brabantia bin for Christmas, because she had 'kept going on' about it. He didn't make that mistake twice, but he also thought he was doing a good thing with the bin because she'd mentioned it so often. All of this comes under the heading 'Communication'. They are a great thriving couple, and the bin incident has gone down in folklore. She will never receive a kitchen appliance as a gift again, however much she'd been harping on about one in the lead-up to Christmas or her birthday.

HUG IT OUT

By midlife you might have been together or been married twenty years or more, like me and Kenny, so you'd hope the communication issue was sorted. Well, it might have been for a few years,

but often it's broken down through busyness or bad habits creep-
ing in – texts and WhatsApps replacing proper chats and time
together, for example. The relationships I have seen cracking in
midlife are the ones who don't seem to have addressed these issues
properly, then they wait for the children to leave home and hope
somehow with the new-found freedom and time available it's going
to magically fix itself. But like the homes we live in, if we don't do
the little repairs along the way, the cracks will become bigger and
eventually the house will fall apart.

How often do you hug your partner? Touch their hand or hold
it? If it's fairly regularly then I am guessing things are quite good
between you. If you don't go in for a little cuddle while the kettle is
boiling, or a peck on the cheek before heading to work, could you
try to add it to your daily life, and see how you both feel? I know
it's busy at breakfast time, but a hug before you go off for the day
takes seconds and when you come in later in the day, your partner
might be in the middle of something, but how long does it take to
kiss them on the lips to say hello, or give them a hug and ask about
their day? We might be talking one minute at both ends of the day.
Two minutes a day, fourteen minutes a week, an hour a month,
if someone said to you when you first met you need to devote an
hour a month to help keep the romance of this relationship alive,
you'd have laughed at how easy the request was.

There are also important health benefits of hugging:

- It's a stress reducer which helps lower blood pressure and
  improve heart health
- Cortisol levels reduce with each cuddle, which can
  improve immunity
- The pleasure hormone oxytocin is released by physical
  touch, which boosts good moods

Trust me, I don't always get this right and I will be told if
I forget these little gestures. If I come in from work and don't

give Kenny a hug, I get a look and later a word in my ear. That's what my partner needs, in the same way I might be more inclined to deliver hugs if I come in and don't trip over fourteen pairs of shoes by the back door – and if he's remembered to turn the outside lights on, he might get an even longer hug. This is our little dance; he knows what makes me feel calm and happy when I come home, and I know he's missed me and needs a bit of physical contact and that he might also then want to tell me all about his day.

That's not to say random hugging doesn't happen around here, of course it does and nobody ever felt worse for being pulled in by their partner and given a reassuring hug, fully clothed in the middle of the day, i.e., not given because they think that there might be sex in the kitchen at the end of it (although if you do have the little moments of touch through the day you might be more likely to have sex later on).

YOUR PRESENCE IS YOUR PRESENT

Kenny has always been one to go a bit overboard at Christmas, and while I love his taste and the choices he makes, it's the random gifts he pops in the stocking that mean more than the expensive handbag or dress he's splashed the cash on. Last year I unwrapped a new iPad cover which had a special feature on it to elevate it, so it was more like working on a laptop or a PC. As I opened it, I could see he was worried, that this could be our 'Brabantia bin' moment. 'I thought this would be really helpful when you are writing at work or travelling,' he said nervously. I loved it – not only is it super helpful to me but I hadn't asked for it or mentioned it, he'd simply noticed how I work and that it would be useful and make my life a little easier. That for me was a true moment of romance. Him wanting to do things that make my life less complicated.

NEGOTIATING THE NIGGLES

Of course, I annoy Kenny, and he annoys me. How can you be together for twenty-four years and not? Couples who say they never argue are either not spending any time together or someone in that relationship is not communicating their truth. Disagreement is healthy, but learning how to do it can take time. What took me a while to convey in our relationship was that I didn't want to win every time; it is not a sporting contest. Because we are both very competitive by nature, Kenny didn't believe me. I did a law degree; formulating the argument and making my points was almost as much fun to me as the outcome. He's an ex-rugby player; he just wanted to put in a verbal big hit. We had to navigate a way to disagree that was somewhere in the middle and learn that sometimes nobody is right: we just had a difference of opinion. When it comes to issues regarding the kids, we always agreed to take those conversations away from the subject matter, so the child in question never saw or heard us argue about them. We agreed to present a united front until we could thrash it out privately later . . . when I then won the argument. I am joking.

And joking might be one of the most important tools you can have in your relationship arsenal. If you can't laugh at yourself, you probably won't be laughing much together. There are times it won't be easy to keep the giggles and fun coming; believe me, there are lots of reasons why it might feel harder to laugh at yourself in midlife. Menopausal symptoms aren't very funny; looking at your face losing more collagen every day, thinning hair, living with stressed hormonal teenagers, dealing with ageing and sick parents and all the other physical challenges we have discussed through the last few chapters do not add up to an award-winning night at the Apollo. But somehow, we have to find the funny because a relationship without fun is just bloody hard work.

The Midpointer View

Actress, documentary maker, TV personality, writer, comedian, and now the holder of an MA in cognitive therapy from Oxford University, Ruby Wax knows how much it takes to keep a relationship on track. 'When we were going down the aisle, I told [husband Ed] I had two husbands before him and that I was mentally ill. So, he was prepared. His dad was a colonel and so he knew about war, and his great-grandfather was in the trenches, so he's trained for mental illness Ed – he's good for emergencies. Not everything's perfect, we have different lives, so we don't see each other that much. He doesn't compete with me. He's not threatened. He likes it when I'm funny. I throw him a laugh once a year and that's enough to keep him. I think it's important to laugh, though, isn't it? That keeps you together longer than a big pair of boobs, doesn't it?'

LOVE CLINIC

I got relationship expert Annabelle Knight on to *The Midpoint* to get some straight talk about all aspects of midlife marriages and relationships. I'd noticed lots of people my age getting a bit bored and fed up with their partner, and quite a few marriages breaking down. With divorce rates rocketing in all age groups, we'll talk about the devastation divorce can bring in midlife in the chapter on loss. But here, in this chapter, we're focused on making love work before it's too late and why we shouldn't all be looking for an upgrade when we have a rough few days, weeks or months with our romantic partner. Might it be that we don't need to throw the baby out with the bath water, but simply address why the person you were once madly in love with is suddenly really annoying you. Like me and Kenny, I'm sure you have your niggles and annoyances – and your partnership sometimes feels stale – so I asked Annabelle the big questions.

How can you save a tired midlife marriage?

'Being able to talk to your partner is key. I talk about communication until I'm blue in the face and I'm often met with eye rolls because every single couple I meet think, Well, of course we communicate; we talk every single day. But real communication involves active listening, honesty and openness. And without those three pillars, you are just talking hot air. With communication, it is about raising issues as and when they arrive so they don't fester, so they don't become something more than what you can handle as a couple. After communication, it's really important to be completely honest with your partner in all aspects of your relationship – and that is everything from your financials and the day-to-day running of your shared lives, to things in the bedroom and things out of the bedroom as well. Your friends, your family . . . Every element needs to be met with complete transparency so that you have a really good chance of making the relationship work in the long term.'

When a relationship is not salvageable, and you move on into the dating wilderness again – which for a lot of people in their forties will be a truly new landscape – how do they face dating again?

'A lot of people don't give themselves enough credit for what they have just been through. A relationship breakdown is a trauma and it needs to be dealt with in such a way that you are ready to come into the dating world afterwards. If you jump in too soon, you end up subliminally seeking out relationships, whether you mean to or not, that are going to fail because you're not actually in the right head space to have a successful relationship. Giving yourself that grieving time and that time to reconnect with yourself, reconnect with what life means to be single, all of those things are really important before someone jumps back into the dating world.'

Does that include having a casual bit of sex with somebody? Should they try celibacy and enjoying their own company?

'I wouldn't necessarily say try to be celibate, but I would say if you're seeking something more meaningful and more long term than just a bit of fun, then definitely give yourself the time. But of course, a one-night stand or a fling can be one of those blocks of building that bridge to your new life. It really depends on the individual, but definitely take your time and think about what it is that you need for yourself in order to move on.'

For those looking for love in midlife, how does dating work now?

'Dating apps with people in their forties and fifties are becoming increasingly popular. We can see data that shows us that the forty-plus age group is one of the most burgeoning age groups for using online dating. A lot of people are trying them, but they prefer dating websites where you get to put a little bit more information in and it's not quite as instant because that instant-ness is a little off-putting for people if you are used to meeting people in a more organic setting and letting relationships grow, whether that's meeting partners at work or through friends. [Dating apps] are very, very in your face; it's, "I'm single, I'm looking for someone, please approach me." And you get micro rejection with dating apps. Every time you match with someone that doesn't match with you, you get a little sad feeling, but every time you match with someone that does match with you, you get a little hit of dopamine. So, it's a little chemical rush either way. With the dating apps, I think if you are not used to that kind of fast-paced and instantaneous dating lifestyle, it might be a little bit of a shock for you. My advice for anyone looking for online dating is to have a look at the different ways you can date online and pick the one that fits in with you the best.'

The Midpointer View

Kelly Cates, the Sky Sport Premier League football anchor, is recently divorced with two young daughters, and is not sure how bothered she is with dating. 'The thought of going on a date and spending an evening with somebody and at the end of it thinking, Well, I don't really like you. I would be so resentful of that, of them taking up my time – bearing in mind, I don't get a chance to see the people I do like very often. Imagine going out with somebody and you sit there halfway through, and you think, God, this guy's an idiot and you've just wasted a babysitter.'

LET'S TALK ABOUT SEX

Statistically, if you enter midlife sexually active, then you are more likely to continue to be sexually active into old age. My midlife friends and acquaintances currently seem to fall into a few distinct different groups when it comes to sex. Is your social circle similar? There are:

- The long-term relationships that still have fairly regular sex
- The long-termers who have all but given up on sex
- The newly divorced singletons who go through a period of fun; sometimes too much fun

- The newly divorced singletons wary of going on a
  dating app
- The longer-term divorced people who, after a period
  of feast and then famine, settle into something like a
  relationship of convenience – friends with benefits, if
  you will
- The divorcees who take on a whole new relationship for
  life and get married again and possibly have more kids

Recognise those groupings? The one I worry about the most are
the longer-termers who aren't having sex any more, because I can't
believe that both sides are equally happy with this arrangement. If
they're both content with finding affection and connection outside
of the bedroom, good for them, but in the longer term I wonder
if there is a partner who is keener to have sex than the other, and
might go elsewhere for their desires to be satisfied.

KEEPING IT UP

Orgasms are good for us – releasing endorphins (to boost your
mood) and oxytocin, that hug hormone which is good for bond-
ing and building intimacy and connection that lasts outside the
bedroom – so we should keep having sex … But when things
have gone a bit stale and you really would rather sit down in front
of Netflix with a cup of tea than get hot and flustered with your
partner of God knows how long, how can you find the motivation?

Having a regular sex life might sound like a trivial wish in the
scheme of bigger health issues that you could be affected by, but
if it's something that is impacting your relationship and personal
happiness then it can have enormous negative ramifications – not
least on your mental well-being. Because of the physical work-out,
connection and feel-good hormones sex releases, regular sexual
activity:

- Boosts immunity
- Improves heart health
- Strengthens the pelvic floor and bladder control
- Relieves headaches
- Helps with other menopausal symptoms and period pain
- Burns calories
- Lowers blood pressure
- Improves sleep
- Reduces stress

... and it's often quite good fun. I've given you a decent list of reasons why it's worth making a bit of effort to keep your sex life going, but the simple truth seems to be use it or lose it.

The Midpointer View

Actor Tamzin Outhwaite shared in our chat on the podcast how she has discovered a confidence and happiness in midlife that she takes into the bedroom with her twenty-years-younger boyfriend. 'I really have never felt sexier, and I think that's because [my boyfriend] somehow gets that about me, that I'm in a stage in my life where I'm really comfortable, I'm happy and I adore him. We have a wonderful time, but if he wasn't around, I wouldn't be in the corner on the floor sliding down walls crying. I would still have my complete life. And he just enhances that and that's what's lovely.' Is it hard being with a younger man when you're in your fifties? 'I feel like everyone around me of this age are sexier, but they're trying much less hard to be sexy. Yes, they're much more relaxed, but they've got a sense of knowing wisdom that's really quite intriguing.'

I asked relationship guru Annabelle Knight how couples who have been together for a chunk of time can keep their sex lives hot and spicy. 'It is quite a difficult subject for a lot of people to tackle,' she admitted, 'but sex is something that we all do, unless you are in a sexless relationship. For the most part, people enjoy being intimate with their partners, but the majority of people don't know how to express their needs, wants and desires because we're very stiff upper lip. We put up and shut up, we lie back and think of England – all those kinds of things that you are met with across the board societally ... But that is changing. People are getting more confident in the bedroom. I love the rise of body positive and sex positive influencers because their message, which a few years ago may have been met with rolled eyes, is now being absorbed by the masses. We see a lot of people deciding, "Actually my sex life isn't quite what I want it to be. It's not terrible, but it's not amazing" – and it can be amazing and you should want amazing and you should strive for amazing. Even if they're not quite at the point where they feel they can speak to their partner, they're at a point with themselves where they know that they want to be able to speak to their partner.'

Annabelle's advice for boosting your sex life

I always say this to my couples: every relationship is completely different. You all have your unique styles, so finding the ways in which you can muddle through together are slightly different for everyone. So, while these are general tips, if there is something that specifically works for you, please don't throw that out of the window. Keep doing that.

- Active transparency is something that can be introduced into a relationship: micromanaging your annoyances, so instead of those problems festering and growing a mountain from a molehill, they're dealt with in the

here and now. They become non-events and because
you are talking to your partner and you have a constant
dialogue going with this active transparency, you have
a much clearer understanding of what drives them and
what ticks them off in a much clearer, much concise
way. You can manage your behaviour better if you know
something you do or some way you behave causes a
negative impact on your partner. You can adjust your
own behaviour and they can adjust theirs, finding that
middle ground and meeting there.

- It's completely normal and natural that we're going to get
  oversaturated with our partner, which is why practising
  mindfulness is so important. If you are so aware of your
  partner and yourself and how that is affecting you in
  the here and now, you can act on that instead of letting
  it fester or trying to repress those feelings because you
  think that's better in the long run. I'm a huge believer
  in grab the bull by the horns when it comes to issues in
  relationships. Anything left can rot and that causes a
  level of toxicity that's very hard to cleanse yourself from.

- If you watch those (sex) scenes in films and think,
  That hasn't happened for me for such a long time, but
  I would like it to happen, there are things you can do
  to implement that. One of the things I love to get my
  couples to do is to write down five sexual scenarios
  that they would love to find themselves in, whether
  that's acts, positions, places, role play. Whatever it is,
  write down five things that you'd love to do. You might
  want to revisit something, but it's a sexual scenario that
  you have a desire for and you get your partner to do
  the same thing and then you just cross-reference lists
  and it's so common that a couple will have a similar
  thing that they both would like to do within those five
  things.

- I get mocked so much because people say there's nothing sexy about planning for sex, but I say plan. It's not sexy but it does ensure that you have sex ... And sex is sexy when you are having it. It only takes a few moments of, 'Oh God, we're doing this again,' before your natural instincts take over and it becomes really enjoyable.
- Remember, sex is like going to the gym. The more you do it, the more you want to do it.

BRINGING SEXY BACK

Let's look at a few positives about being in midlife when it comes to your sexual relationships. You know what you like, and if you are in a longer-term relationship, you have hopefully learnt how to communicate that to your partner, but if things get a bit stale you will also feel confident enough to say, 'Can we try something new?'

If you have children, they are either going or gone from the family home and you might feel less restricted to the 'quick one' before lights go out. Even if they still live at home, by now they shouldn't be hanging out in it all day, nor should they be appearing at the foot of your bed in the middle of the night. So, you can have daytime sex again! I know my kids will kill me for over-sharing, but it's a plus point of being empty-nesters. And if you are my local mates, please don't let this put you off popping by for coffee unannounced, this is all theory and not necessarily regular practice.

By this stage, you are well over the hang-ups you may have had about your body in your twenties. So especially if you are embarking on new sexual relationships, take that confidence forwards and remember if you are dating similar types, they are probably feeling exactly the same.

Whatever your relationship status is as you read this chapter, think about what your relationships have taught you about those you choose to love and have sex with, and about yourself. Remember: your romantic relationships should be whatever you want and need them to be. A fulfilling love and sex life looks different on everyone. Don't share judgements on anyone else's relationships unless asked for them, and don't let unwanted opinions get in the way of what works for you.

Of course, your sex life might have slowed down well before midlife and you might be happy with that, but as always, the midlife can throw up some physical challenges related to our changing hormones which affect our sexual appetite and comfort. I want to emphasise, there is no right or wrong level of libido – no box to tick or number to hit – but you might be remembering what your libido was like as a twenty-something in a steady relationship, or as a newly married person, and feel you are now lacking or that something is wrong. Try this: think of a period in your life when your sex life was at its healthiest, and you'll have an idea of what was normal for you. I do think some people remember the past differently; if you were only having sex once a month in your thirties it might be unrealistic to expect it three times a week in your fifties with the same partner.

Childbirth and parenting, cancer therapy, depression, hormone drops, anxiety, exhaustion and immune disorders can all cause a decrease in sexual appetite. You may have experienced this feeling before in your life. You might have already discussed it with your GP, but if you haven't it really is worth talking about what your options are. In my opinion all GP practices should have a female health specialist, but the chances are you won't have that option, so find out from your practice receptionist who is most qualified and ask to see that person. If they can't suggest anyone, I would respond that you want to be referred or change practice.

The Midpointer View

Davina McCall had some thoughts on libido and midlife sex scenarios that she shared on the podcast. 'What I think is really interesting is when we are in our late twenties, early thirties, biology and human nature are telling us to find a mate to procreate. I mean the biological clock – mine was so freaking loud. I was like, "Inseminate me, give me a baby," out there hunting for a father. I think in later life, if we are talking midpoint, when you are past having babies, biologically you are not looking to procreate, you are looking for something completely different. You are looking for a connection on a different level. Physically and mentally, but without biologically going, "You have to impregnate me," it's a different form of connection. I feel like the older you get, the freer you are with your physique and your body; you're not ashamed or embarrassed about your lumps and bumps any more. I always say I haven't got the body of a twenty-year-old any more, but I love the body that I've got.'

SEXUAL HEALING

When I finally realised I was experiencing perimenopausal symptoms, one of the boxes I ticked was a drop-off in libido. I had been prepared to accept it as a symptom of ageing and being in a very long-term relationship. Maybe that's what naturally happens to everyone, I surmised. But when I understood it was part of a bigger picture, and I could possibly change it, it was an enormous relief. It wasn't my main motivation to take HRT, but the impact was almost immediate, within a week. I still fancied my husband,

and continuing to be sexually active and enjoying it – not just dutifully turning up – was important to us. My kids will kill me if I say any more than that.

As we age there might be other reasons why a sexual relationship might not be possible, and for the best part of a year Kenny and I faced some of those challenges. After his prostatectomy, which I wrote about in Chapter 8, we knew the chances of Kenny having immediate functionality were very slim and he'd probably have to take pills for a while. He had a plan which he worked out with his urologist and that involved us trying, while knowing it might take a while to 'work'. We had to work out other ways of enjoying sexual relations until that functionality returned. Again, for the kids' sake, you can use your imagination on that one.

There are many other factors which can affect erectile functionality in midlife – carrying excess weight, depression, diabetes and heart disease, to name a few – and there are a range of medications which can help. But what's clear from the kind of diseases that affect erectile function is that eating well, being healthy and maintaining a good weight are all going to mean you are more likely to stay fully 'functioning'.

MIDPOINT ACTION POINTS

- Good love lives and sex lives all come down to communication: check how you talk to others, and to yourself. Don't speak down to anyone, including you. Talk openly, honestly, kindly and clearly to those you love about what you want and need, and listen in return.
- If you find yourself suddenly single at midlife, before you look for love again, try to reflect honestly on what went wrong in the past and your part in it. Get yourself

healthy before you try to place yourself in a healthy relationship.

- There is nothing shameful about sex. It's natural, needed by most of us, and should be lots of fun. Speak to your friends, speak to your partner, speak to your doctor, if anything is worrying you or feels different or strange.
- There is no happy ever after. Keeping relationships happy and healthy requires constant love, work and attention. Everyone has imperfections, bad days, annoying habits, but if the good outweighs the bad, they are worth putting up with because long-term love really can be a many-splendoured thing.

13 FAMILY

Family is a life jacket in the stormy sea of life.

J. K. ROWLING

When my mum turned fifty, I was twenty-seven years old and had just got engaged to my now husband. When I turned fifty, my kids were seventeen and about to do their A levels. One of my best friends is fifty next spring and will have the eldest of her four children in his second year at university and the youngest in Year 2 at primary school, only seven years old. I guess my point is that your kids could be any age when you hit the midlife. You might also have a blended family, with some kids leaving home and finding their feet on their own in the world, while the younger kids are still under your feet and with you twenty-four/seven. There is no normal in midpoint parenting, but interestingly the average age of a woman giving birth to her first child in the UK today is 29.6 years, not dramatically different to the average age in 1938 which was 29 years old. I guess we are still working on the basis that the average family will be experiencing children leaving home for university or work as the older adults in the house hit midlife, which is my scenario.

It's often noted that Mother Nature was playing a cruel trick reducing the hormones in the female at such a rapid rate around the time the same hormones are going into overdrive in her teenage progeny. For teenagers and mothers that can be an interesting time, and in our house, I found the best way to deal with it was to be totally open about the menopause and what its symptoms were and why I felt I needed to take HRT. I was then able to comfortably explain why their own hormonal changes might be responsible for emotionally charged moments or a spot break-out or PMS bloating. There's been a lot of hormone upheaval in our house over the last decade. Lois's first period arrived while I was away presenting *Match of the Day*. Kenny dealt with it brilliantly, although she saved the rant for me when I got home. 'I have this every month for the next forty years! It's awful, Mother Nature should have worked out a better way by now,' she cried as I gave her a cuddle. I nodded in agreement.

The Midpointer View

Tess Daly described on the podcast what most working mothers feel, especially when we reach midlife as we have our own stuff to deal with, even perhaps looking after our parents, on top of our kids. 'My biggest challenge is keeping all the plates in the air as a working mum. Being there for any of the special school-related occasions; being there whenever my kids need me – and they need you more than ever, I think, as they get older – but also doing the job that I love that defines me as a person, that I enjoy and I don't want to sacrifice. Just trying to strive for that eternal balance we're all trying to straddle.'

EMPTY-NESTERS

Having twins, I was always slightly dreading the day they both decided to go to university at the same time. From the noise and busyness of a hectic family home, how would we deal with quietness, the tidiness and space? Thankfully we got a reprieve. Our son Reuben did head off, albeit to become a rugby player not a student per se, so I joked that we got him off the pay roll! Our daughter Lois decided to have a gap year to focus on her sporting passion, horses, and to pay for her travel plans (travelling with a horse is expensive) so she'll be home for a while working. Lois is kindly easing us into the empty nest.

The night we dropped Reuben off at his new home, which is only ninety minutes away, Lois decided to spend the evening at her boyfriend's house, which was bad timing from her – we could have done with the remaining child at home to ease the pain. So, having stocked Reuben's new fridge and made sure his bed was made up and his TV and internet worked, we arrived back to our now eerily quiet family home.

It was a gorgeous June evening, I started making dinner and when I went outside to set the table, I found Kenny watering plants and watering his own cheeks with his tears; and for that first week, Kenny could talk about little else than missing Reuben. I missed him too, but I was also proud of him working and training hard at a sport he loved, and knew we'd all get used to our new situation. Reuben was confused by how his dad felt, and having to deal with all the change thrown at him, too. He saw his mates having their fun post-A-level summer while he was getting 'beasted' in pre-season training. He loves rugby, and felt elated to be able to call playing it his job, but the reality of being a responsible adult and acknowledging that, unlike his mates who were students, this was him 'gone' hit him hard. He wouldn't be coming home for a reading week, or the Christmas holidays or Easter holidays for weeks at a time.

He did find a rhythm and worked out he could get back by train on his days off, which thrilled us obviously. 'I'd rather chill out here with you guys,' he told us on one trip home. He missed the dogs, and he missed our company, which was a revelation. He was becoming an adult, and appreciating the life and the home we'd built for him and his sister. It was a lovely feeling.

They spend their teenage years pushing boundaries and buttons and telling you they can't wait to leave and then almost immediately realise they are not quite as grown up as they thought they were. I was glad I was dealing with this emotional maelstrom in a better place than I had been a few years before when the perimenopausal symptoms were hitting hard. The moodier, more anxious me might not have coped so well with these changes. I quickly realised that the empty nest is both a triumph ... and a slightly exaggerated concept. A triumph because what most of us are working towards for eighteen years is to produce children who want to pursue passions and interests and have the confidence to do so. If they want to head into the world to be educated or to work, then that is a brilliant achievement. It is also increasingly unlikely that the nest is ever truly empty. Our children cannot even imagine being able to rent on their own, let alone buy a home, at the moment or for the foreseeable. I see the birds flying in and out of this nest for a good few years to come.

The Midpointer View

Football legend Phil Neville is like me, and dreading an empty nest ... while looking forward to the freedom, too. 'I think about it every day,' he said during our podcast conversation. 'I want [my son] to go and enjoy his life, but with my daughter, there's that protection of my little baby. She's my little girl. She is my weakness; she definitely is. I think every time I drop her off at school, She might not be here in another year's time. Dads and the daughters have a relationship that's like no other. And I suppose my wife will be thinking the same about Harvey – she doesn't want him to move out. I'm looking forward to the empty nest – I want my wife back a little bit, you know? I mean, the school pick-up times, the meal times. I think just before we had children, we were like twenty-one, twenty-two, so there were so many things we wanted to do. We wanted to travel, we wanted to go to places. There're so many places that I want to explore that she wants to explore, maybe our children can come with us, maybe they don't, but we can rewind back. They can dip in and out of our lives, but ultimately, me and my wife – we're inseparable.'

THE BENEFIT OF A NEW RHYTHM

Having said that, when the school timetable stopped for ever it was like ripping off a set of handcuffs. Interestingly, I am not getting up any later, as I had previously fantasised. I quite like being an early riser now that I have had fifteen years of 6.15 a.m. alarm calls. But remember, parents a few years behind, who fear their children growing up, there are lots of pluses:

- I like the feeling at the other end of the day that I am not rushing back from whatever I am doing to get meals ready or help with lifts to sports events.
- The day feels longer, but in a positive way. Kenny and I both feel more productive. Even though my kids have not finished school at 3.30 p.m. for a few years now and

they have been at schools with buses, there was a legacy
from the early years of primary education of feeling
like I had to try to wrap up projects on the days I was
working from home at 3 p.m.
- There is a freedom to do more of the things I want to do,
so I might finish at 3 p.m. but then go and play nine holes
of golf or have a facial or carry on working if I want to.
- Then there was the quick trip to Portugal in September.
I don't think we have ever been away in September
because pre-children Kenny was playing professional
rugby and we were dictated to by the season.
- A few years ago, I realised that I was going to have time
for my old hobbies soon. As a full-time worker, full-time
mum and full-time wife, I had let the fun hobbies slide.
I still made time to be fit but the hedonism of spending
a few hours on a golf course just didn't sit well with my
busy life, it left me feeling guilty not relaxed.

All of this change and space does mean that there is more time
to think and make plans. If you haven't looked ahead and arrive
at this junction without any planning, it could be a bit of a shock.
You will probably have a totally different list of neglected hobbies
and ambitions that you might fancy picking up. My advice is don't
wait until the day your last child finishes their A levels, get yourself
ready for the space.

Of course, not all late-forties parents are looking forward to the
freedom of an empty nest. My friend and colleague Denise Lewis
had her fourth baby at forty-seven years old, and there have been
quite a few well-known women giving birth in the back end of the
forties and beyond: Victoria Coren Mitchell, Naomi Campbell and
Tana Ramsay, to name a few. I am envious and also relieved it's not
me in equal measure. I love babies but I am fairly knackered with
teenagers, work and the menopause; but I guess it's a mindset and
there are also a lot of positives about having children a bit later.

RAISING TEENAGERS

Parenting never gets easier ... it just gets different. Mothering my teens has been a shock for me: I thought the nappy changing and sleepless nights of the baby and toddler years would be the hard graft; but what I've learnt is just as I was getting older and more tired, hitting my midpoint, my teens needed me mentally and emotionally more than ever. Parenting in this period of life is something that Caitlin Moran touched on in her book *More Than a Woman*, and she agreed the teenage years can be tricky for a midlife parent. 'That's a big old blow, when you get to your middle age, and you thought it was going to get easier and it's not. It's like you *really* have to turn up and put the hours in when they're a teenager.'

It's true. Parenting, whatever stage, whatever age, doesn't get easier, it just gets different. Hang in there ... but how? Caitlin came on the podcast and shared invaluable advice for other parents in midlife who are dealing with teenagers – and I especially loved her ideas around how we should engage our kids in world news, while protecting them, at this crucial time. The world can feel like a horrible, scary, dangerous place, so I wanted to know from this wise woman how she had conversations, as a family, about the state of the world that wasn't all doom and gloom.

'Whatever your political persuasion, whatever your household, I think everybody thinks this is a fairly unhopeful age – environmental, political, economic – and you have these conversations around the table with your friends, then suddenly realise there's a little pair of eyes in the corner looking really scared. And then what we do, thinking that we're going to make it better as adults, is we go, "But don't worry because your generation is amazing. You kids are going to be amazing. You are going to save the world. So don't worry." And we think that's a compliment and that we're making them feel better, but of course it isn't! It's huge pressure.

The kids are just hearing, "Save Mummy and Daddy. We don't know what to do." And the other thing we do often is we go, "In the end, it doesn't matter how you do at school or what you look like, or any of these things, Mummy and Daddy just want you to be happy" ... again thinking that that's a really kind thing to say, but a kid's just hearing, "Okay, so I have to be happy for you? If you saw me being sad or worried or anxious, I failed you?"

'Often when we think we're being kind, or useful, or empowering our children, we actually aren't. And it is such an anxious age at the moment. We have to find a way to make them less anxious and make them feel that Mummy and Daddy are in charge of this, and we are going to do something about it, and we're not leaving it to the next generation. I had a friend at *The Times* who, when her children reached teenage years, she resigned from her desk job and I was like, "What? Why?" Because I had very little kids and she said, "This is where they really need you." It's a specialist job being a parent in the teenage years. When they're younger, they just need someone to stop them falling down the stairs and hug them, but in the teenage years, you become like a professional psychiatrist and guide to adult life, and teenagers working in a very specific way will feel sad or bad about something for ages and then there's a two-minute window in maybe a month where they'll be ready to talk to you about it. And that's it. If you're not there for that conversation, if you're not driving them somewhere or just slumped around watching telly together, if you're not there when they want to turn to you and talk, you can miss that window for months. I didn't realise how just finely balanced and finely tuned it was, and you just have to be around.'

PARENTING YOUR PARENTS

The other big change to family life that occurs for those in the midlife is that often they have to start caring for their parents – the roles held previously in everyone's lives are reversed. I am sure you have heard of the expression 'sandwich generation': midlifers who still have dependants at home in the form of teenagers but also have ageing parents they are caring for and often financially providing for too. I have had a small taste of this sandwich life: my dad was in and out of hospital or needing a lot of care and attention for a few years. Thankfully his health seems to have stabilised and he now has someone who visits him a few times a week to make sure he's taking his medication and looking after himself. I think the health stabilising and the carer starting are inextricably linked. We live over two hundred miles away from him so it wasn't possible to give that daily attention he needed; we always seemed to be dashing up when there was a crisis. Now I can call his carer and make sure she's happy with what is going on or tell her he needs a doctor's appointment for a blood test and she will take him. I also managed to get a Health and Welfare Lasting Power of Attorney (LPA) in place when his health was poor as I was concerned he wouldn't be in a position to make good decisions. As his health has improved, we haven't needed to use it, but getting it in place has been a good move. If you think that might be on the horizon for you – that you might need to make big health decisions for a loved one – then applying for an LPA is a good move and can save you stress down the line.

These days my brother takes my dad to watch Leeds United play or takes him out for a meal and between him and my mum, whom he is divorced from but lives close to, we seem to have things under control. You don't ever imagine when you are a kid that one day you'll be looking after your fit, strong, robust parents, but that is the reality for many people as their parents' physical and mental health declines.

Very often, you have a career, kids and a marriage but somehow you are going to have to find time to add caring for your parents into that mix and that is not an easy ask. Even if your kids have flown the nest, or you're happily single and have no other dependants, it's still a big undertaking and can lead to a mental stress you didn't see coming. If you have siblings, it's important to keep the lines of communication open and honest; sometimes it's tough to admit the frailty of a parent but you all want what is best. There will be times when one of you has more time to take up the slack and times when the other sibling might be open to a bit more of the heavy lifting, but if you can share the care, you'll all feel better mentally and physically. It's never too soon to chat to a parent about how they see their future care and what they'd ideally like to happen. Whatever happens and however successful we are in balancing the sandwich of caring for children and parents, we are likely to lose our parents in the midlife period unless they had us exceptionally young, and no matter how much we recognise their mortality it is still something that can side swipe our sense of who we are and what is our place in the world.

MIDPOINT ACTION POINTS

- They're paying attention to you, your kids – and actions speak louder than words. Show them love, show others kindness, take good manners out into the world and to work.
- As my *Midpoint* guests have stressed, communication really is key. Your kids, especially your pre-teens and teens, might not want to talk very often, but when they do, try to be there to listen ...
- Because before you know it, they'll be gone. Living in an empty nest can be brutal at first – you'll miss the noise, the humour, the gossip, even the mess (maybe!). Instead of focusing on what has gone, focus on all the new freedom you have – no more parent-übering, less washing to do, more time for friends and holidays.

- Do the best you can for your parents when they need you, but don't run yourself into the ground – you'll be no good to anyone. Talk to your parents about how they see their future care; discuss it openly, and share the load with siblings if you can. You must look after your own stress levels at this tricky time, so do ask for help and find support within the community.

14 FRIENDS

Lots of people want to ride with you in the limo, but what you want is someone who will take the bus with you when the limo breaks down.

OPRAH WINFREY

Friends are more important than we perhaps give them credit for. Much attention is paid to romantic love, parental love, self-love . . . but research has proven that one of the best things we can do for our mental and physical health is to stay active and social with a group of people who make us feel happy and alive. Professor Rose Anne Kenny is the founding principal investigator of the Irish Longitudinal Study on ageing, and the author of *Age Proof: The New Science of Living a Longer and Healthier Life*. She explained on the podcast how those who live in 'Blue Zone' areas of the world, a term used to describe the places where people generally live the longest, have shown that strong and varied relationships can actually slow down our biological ageing.

'There was one researcher who spent time in Sardinia and she went into the kitchen of a 102-year-old man and sat there, and he was up and dressed and three generations were living in the house, and the kitchen was fronting onto the main road. She sat down to interview him . . . [and] she didn't get a word in edgeways, almost all day, because everybody who was passing popped in to say hello to him. And then the other three generations were moving up and down, popping in and out to the kitchen, chatting to him all the time. She hadn't a moment. And it really occurred to her, "Wow, I mean this is like a railway station and this person is constantly being stimulated by different people, different conversations, different reflections, peppered by meals." She said it was a real eye opener for her. And I think that that is one of the secrets the Blue Zones have in common. They all have social engagement, social connectedness and variety in whatever is stimulating them. Of course, we don't all, unfortunately, live on a small cobbled street in Sardinia, so we need to think of creative ways that we can actually shape our lives with that sort of fun.'

Why are busy social lives good for us as we get older?

- They give purpose
- They boost creativity
- Laughter is the best medicine. That well-known expression has now translated into true science at a biological level
- Sharing and talking through our worries reduces stress, and reduces adrenalin and cortisol. In Sardinia, people meet once a day for a chat, usually in the afternoon, usually with a glass of wine. There are lots of experiments from university student groups right through to older age groups to show that a problem shared really *is* a problem halved in terms of biological impacts.

MATES FOR LIFE

I thought I was happy to close the list on friends for a while there in my late thirties; I subconsciously wore an invisible sign or gave off a vibe which said, *I am full on friends now; sorry, no more room here.* I wasn't unfriendly, just a bit unsociable. When I look back and reflect, I think a few different factors were at play. I was physically exhausted, work was hectic, we kept renovating homes and moving, the children had busy social and school lives and it was that phase of parenting where you seem to suddenly be part of loads of events and WhatsApp groups that you didn't really need to join but life is all about making the kids happy so you go along with it.

You find yourself hanging out on a Friday evening with a lot of people you don't really know, the parents of your kids' friends, when the people you have known for years, whom you love and miss dearly, don't get to see you because they live twenty miles away and your socialising becomes quite local because you need a babysitter and don't want to waste hours of time travelling and just don't have the energy. At this point of my busy parenting life, sleep was more important to me than society. I was forever doing sleep mathematics when we received a social invitation: If we go there and leave at midnight, we won't be home until 1 a.m. and so not into bed until at least 1.15 a.m. then up at 6.30. You can see how I got the nickname 'Fun Sponge' from my kids.

I did meet some cool and interesting people through the children, but then I already knew cool and interesting people, and I didn't see them enough. I tried hard to make time for my long-serving mates and then there were the mates Kenny and I had acquired as a couple, but if they didn't have kids at the same age or stage big family gatherings wouldn't always work out as intended – there'd be either bored pre-teens asking when they could go home or some wild toddlers demanding the attention of wine-swilling adults – and time together wasn't as idyllic as we'd hoped it would be. We did just enough to keep the connections alive – and good friends understand everyone goes through different phases – but I missed them.

Yes, maintaining a social life or friendship circle when you're a parent is complicated. I'd keep our socialising to an evening – but not on a school night, of course – which then limited it to the weekends, and then once the kids started doing sport and getting up early on Saturdays and Sundays themselves . . . the effort to go out on a Saturday seemed enormous. In this period, Kenny and I had to set the bar very high. 'Are you getting married?' 'No.' 'Well then, sorry I can't make it.' I'm almost not joking.

These times are what we call our Strictly Years, where we hunkered down at home on a Saturday night with the kids and the TV on, which was lovely but not very sociable. My mum, who hasn't chosen to have a Saturday night in since 1965, would call me around 5 p.m. every Saturday and ask, 'Are you out tonight?' Then on hearing the negative response, she'd sound desperately disappointed for us. I think in her eyes we were neglecting our social lives. But we weren't: we were adapting to what was needed of us, and what we could physically and mentally handle.

Being sociable is tiring. I suppose what I am trying to say is that friends and support groups that you create or join in your life change and morph for various reasons as you go through each decade and some people will last the test of time and others won't, but that's not a bad thing either. It doesn't have to be a dramatic ending. Some friends come into your life because they are what you need at that time – I'm thinking particularly of work colleagues who are good for a moan with in the pub after hours, or the school mums who keep you posted on World Book Day and have a giggle with you at sports days. When you're in a different job, or your kids have left school, you might not see them very much, if at all, but they were good friends when it mattered, and you should always think of them fondly – and without guilt you're no longer in each other's pockets. That's life.

The Midpointer View

Brian O'Driscoll, rugby legend, thinks women are more sussed about the importance of friendships than men. 'I had a conversation the other day with two of my wife's friends who were over for a takeaway, and we were chatting and one of them mentioned how, just before she got married, her dad said, "The really important thing that's going to keep your relationship together is continuing having your own individual relationship with your friends; don't become just a unit together." And she said that's really fuelled her over ten years of marriage. I live the other side of the city than a lot of my friends that I grew up with and I talk to them, but I've got young kids, I've been busy with other things, and you get into this comfort zone of, Ah, we'll be fine. We'll pick up now in a while. You do have to constantly work on relationships and get out the comfort zone. I met with old teammates for a walk the other day. It's kind of weird, seeing three grown men walking down the street, going for a forty-five-minute walk, taking up the whole pathway, you know, but it was lovely to get out and just catch up. It's well and good chatting on the phone, but you don't have that interaction – you don't get the body language, being able to see someone's awkwardness and then asking a supportive second question and so on. It's definitely something I have to be conscious of because I'm very happy in my own company.'

SOCIAL WORK

My social skills picked up when we moved out of London. I had to join in more because I didn't know anyone and then one day, I was picked up by an incredible group of women who spotted I was floundering a bit in my new rural surroundings. They were a very eclectic bunch brought together through geography more than long-term ties and children – the friendships had not been exclusively predicated on having kids at the same school. Our conversations rarely strayed into classroom chatter, or child comparison. It was revelatory to me, because in my early forties as I was then I was being welcomed into a whole new established friendship group with really interesting, clever, funny women. A few years before this, the exhausted me would have turned down the initial invite to go to dinner in the first place.

For many of us, there has often been a natural culling and curating of friendship groups by the landmark fiftieth birthday, which is a time that focuses the mind, not least if you are hosting an event or party to mark the occasion. One of my recently acquired but loveliest girlfriends wanted to host a weekend for me at her second home in Cornwall, which could sleep sixteen. I got to sixteen quite easily; I could certainly have asked a few others, but I was equally sure that those who didn't come whom I class as mates would not be offended. Seeing this amazing group of women together at dinner one night was truly one of my proudest moments. From the two at the table whom I met at eleven years old, to my local mates who came into my life ten years ago when we moved out of London, there was a mix of many stages, ages and areas of life, and they all got along so well, or they were pretending to for my benefit; it was a beautiful time I'll never forget. We had a painting class, swam in a cold sea, jumped into beachside saunas to warm up, did Pilates, danced, and went on windy walks to long lunches. I could not have been happier, doing my favourite things with these amazing women. We immediately planned what our commune would look like and when we were all planning to move in.

The Midpointer View

The wonderful Tamzin Outhwaite always seems to have really valued her female friends above and beyond. I asked her why they were so important to her. 'I'm kind of having a bit of a love affair with myself and definitely my female friends. Oh, they got me through so many dark times. But also, it's not having people there just for the low times. I really think it's important to be able to celebrate each other properly as well. What I love about the friends I have is their willingness to celebrate you as well as be there for you. And I feel like I love celebrating them when they achieve amazing things.'

I realise I am now in a phase of life where I have a bit more time and I want to make the effort with the friends I have; I don't want to let any of them slide away. But that's not to say that my door is shut to new ones. I want to hear what younger people think and try not to live in a silo; I don't want to only hear opinions which are the same as mine, as comforting as that might be. I love it when my teenagers bring their mates round and I hear their thoughts on the world and their cultural perspectives.

This instinctively feels like the way for a better, healthier life beyond The Midpoint, and the empirical evidence also suggests that it's the best way to age. In the five 'Blue Zones' of the world which have communities identified as places where people live longer than average, and many to one hundred, one of the key commonalties was social engagement. The old people kept on being socially active and with multi generations. So, if you are thinking of pulling down the friendship shutters in midlife you might want to think again.

However, what is lovely about midlife confidence is that you don't tolerate people who make you feel anything less than great. The people pleasers among us may find it more of a challenge to edit friends, but we can all agree that time is precious so we need to be a bit more selective about who we choose to give our energy and loyalty to.

The Midpointer View

Sharleen Spiteri is over wasting time on people who don't deserve it, something she sees as a benefit of reaching midlife. 'There's a great freedom that comes with getting older [which] is … you properly actually don't give a shit. I don't need to make any friends. That acceptance of, like, They don't like me. It's fine. You know when you're younger, you're a bit like, Oh God. Now you just go, I don't care. They don't like me, whatever. Move on.'

BFFs?

In her book *Friendaholic: Confessions of a Friendship Addict*, author Elizabeth Day confessed to spending much of her twenties and thirties outsourcing her sense of self to other people and trying to please everyone. She shared with me her advice on creating healthy social connections, and not letting bad friendships take over your life.

How do you know if you should or could be friends with someone?

'Be aware of how a person makes you feel after you've had an interaction with them and then act accordingly. You don't have to verbalise your boundaries. You can just choose to step back and be a bit quieter. And sometimes we all need to do that to protect our mental health. One of the things that I think is really helpful to do is before you decide to be friends with someone, there's a difference between being friendly and choosing to have a friendship. So, when you're in the early stages of being friendly with a mum at the school gates, or someone you met around the water cooler at work, or someone in a yoga class, it's really important to work out what they're expecting of a friendship and what your metric of friendship is.'

Is The Midpoint a good time for a friend detox?

'Yes. It was the midpoint of my life [when I had a detox] and I just thought, Where am I spending my time? And because I had this hangover of people-pleasing, generally if someone asked me to do something, I'd say yes because I'd want to please them. Which is actually a very arrogant thing to say, to believe egotistically that you're that important to them. My closest friends never put those demands on my time, they were so considerate, and therefore I'd end up not seeing them as much, but I actually wanted to see them. They were the really nurturing ones. There's definitely a rebalancing. And I would say it was a mutual detox, actually, because at the point that you start to feel a friendship is more harmful than healing, the chances are that the other person feels that too. I discovered I was able for the first time ever to have a mature friendship ending, where we both expressed that to each other, and it felt so much better than what we often do, which is just fall out of people's lives without an explanation.'

How many friends do we need?

'There is an incredible scientific study done by [British biological anthropologist] Robin Dunbar, who came up with a number called Dunbar's Number of 150, which is the number of connections that a human brain can cope with. Beyond that, we sort of lose our connection points. He finessed this idea and made it into a series of friendship layers, and in your innermost layer he says, you can have up to five really intimate friendships. If you fall in love or you have kids, that will cost you two of those friendships because the amount of time that we need to put into a friendship to make it meaningful, to make it a really close friendship, a 4-a.m.-phone-call friendship, that requires hours. I find that so interesting and actually quite liberating.'

FRIENDSHIP CIRCLES

Dr Pixie McKenna has learnt a lot in the midlife about who she wants around her. She talked to me about quieting down the noise of busy social groups, and letting go of friends who drain and not caring about if you fit in with the in-crowd. That's part of the greatest wisdom ageing gives you – having the confidence to get rid of the loud or unhealthy, and just focus on the good people you have around you. 'I'm not going to waste any time with ... a circle of friends or ... a lifestyle. Be true to yourself. I think that comes through experience. I probably would've just gone along with things that have happened to me because I was just too shy or didn't know better, but you've got to trust in the years that you've been down on this earth, it means something. Whatever your experience has been is shaping the individual that you are today. A bit of self-trust and listening to that inner voice, which I think guides us all and we sometimes just put a mute over it, we need to open that up and listen to it [when it comes to friendships].'

The Midpointer View

If you don't want to make lots of friends in the midlife, or even keep many, that's fine, too — as long as you're happy and have connections elsewhere, like in a strong family unit — just ask footballer Phil Neville. 'I don't have many friends. I don't want many friends. Sir Alex Ferguson used to say to us, "You only need six friends in your life. The ones that are going to carry your coffin." It was a real Scottish thing he used to say because he didn't like entourages around us. So, he'd say, "Look, just get six friends around you. They're the ones that are going to go to the grave with you." So, I've never been one to have lots of friends. I've probably got two or three friends that are real, real friends. And then outside of that, I just cast aside people. I don't really take that many people on, but obviously the boys, Gary, Nicky, Becks and Giggs, are my close friends. They're almost like my brothers. And, I don't see them at all now, obviously [we have] WhatsApp groups, and stuff like that, but they're getting on with their lives.'

His wife does not approve of his anti-friend mindset. 'It's a constant battle with Julie. I've had to adapt and be flexible because she was brought up in an open house [where] their gates were always open.' He has one ally at home, though. 'My son is just like me. He hates anyone coming to the house. For his eighteenth, he didn't want a party, he just went out with my brother Gary for his first drink. I said, "Do you want to take your friends?" No. "I'll just go out with Uncle Gary."'

MIDPOINT ACTION POINTS

- Not having any friends is bad for your health so do try to be social … But fascinatingly, having too many friends is also bad for your health and can lead to higher incidences of depression. Find the happy medium of people who love you, and you trust, and are there to celebrate and commiserate the ups and downs of The Midpoint with you.
- You don't have to do your social life as a duo with your partner. My husband's got a lot of male friends, they are his mates, I'm not particularly friendly with the wives. There's nothing wrong with them, we just don't hang out. He has nights where he just sees them, which I think is great. I love that. They're not part of my friendship group. He seems to just have an infinite amount of time to keep pulling people in!
- Elizabeth Day has a great metaphor that friendships can be either active volcanoes, they have an active part to play in your life, or dormant, but they forever change the landscape that you find yourself in, and who's to say that a dormant volcano won't become active in your life again? Be grateful for all the people you've been lucky enough to call a friend through your ages, stages and phases. Cherish them in the moment, and cherish the memories you made together.

15 LOSS

You gain strength, courage, and confidence by every experience in which you really stop to look fear in the face ... You must do the things which you think you cannot do.

ELEANOR ROOSEVELT

When Elliott Jaques first published his academic paper on the midlife crisis, one of the key points he recognised in the psyche of his case studies was the realisation that they were over half-way through their life and had come face to face with their own mortality. He uncovered that whether you navigate this period of transitioning from young to old successfully – or not – would be determined by, among other things, your acceptance of death. But how can you really be sure you accept death until you are faced with it? Or how can you know if you're strong enough to handle any kind of loss until it knocks on your door? In this chapter, we'll focus on two areas of loss that push us into dark corners of grief in The Midpoint: death and divorce.

THE DEATH OF A LOVED ONE

Having been through the death of a younger sibling (my brother was fifteen when he suddenly died in 1992), I have spent the last thirty years thinking I was much more accepting in my attitude to death than I actually am. My unpreparedness hit home last year when I attended two funerals for parents of my children's friends in the space of a month. To see the spouses and children left behind so bereft, and teenage friends crying and mourning for their mate and for themselves, left me floored.

We are never prepared, no matter what the age of the person we lose or how old we are when we lose them. Not fully. Both individuals were in their fifties, one knew she was dying, the other was sudden. Neither death was better than the other. Both have missed out on seeing their children fly into adulthood; both left partners they had great plans for big adventures with, and between them they left six children who will miss their guidance, love and support for eternity. I felt sick for them all. I felt grateful I was travelling home from each wake with my husband but also mindful that I am almost certainly closer to the end than the beginning.

Attitudes to grief are vastly different depending on where you are on the planet. Being tearful seven years after a death would be accepted as normal in Egypt, while in the US you would be seeing a psychiatrist for grief disorder. This chapter will not tell you how to grieve, or how to make the pain go away, but it may give you an insight into how some of my guests and experts on *The Midpoint* have accepted their own immortality or dealt with the loss of a loved one.

The Midpointer View

Writer and comedian Matt Lucas learnt a lot through loss. His dad died very suddenly at the age of fifty-two, perhaps giving Matt an appreciation for growing older, and a wisdom in midlife that is helping him accept things he cannot change. 'Things get harder, but a lot of things get easier. In a nice way, not worrying so much about what other people think, not trying to constantly appease people. And the longer you are around, the more experience you have, the more you learn. You see the signs, you know, you are less likely to make the same mistakes again, I guess, because you've already made them. Well, I have. I try not to take myself too seriously and I try not to catastrophise too much if something's going wrong. I try not to start worrying about all the things that are going to go wrong as a consequence of that going wrong – because often they don't. And I remind myself that most people are essentially good.'

TIME TO SAY GOODBYE

Attending a funeral tends to focus the mind and recently, over a particular period of twelve months, I had been to four funerals – the two friends mentioned above, my grandma who was ninety-two years old and one of Kenny's best friends, who was also in his early fifties and who had died from the horrific disease MND. My grandma's death was not a shock, but it was painful; she was the matriarch of our family, the glue that joined us together, and a wonderful woman whom we would all miss. But strangely the other three deaths felt even closer to home: we had shared interests and passions, children of similar ages, and life for all of us should have been entering the fun, freeing phase as the youngest of our collective broods were about to finish school. I have always had a sense of urgency since my brother died; once again it was heightened. Time, I felt, was not on my side.

When my brother died the feeling was of wanting to achieve great things to honour him; he'd missed out on adulthood so I would live it for him, I would put maximum effort into everything I did. I was pure *carpe diem*. These recent deaths, though, have left me feeling more reflective about 'who' I am, not what I do, and maybe that's what Elliott Jaques was nodding towards. I have worked out over the years that you can't seize the day every single day – that's exhausting for you and everyone around you. The eulogies at these fifty-something funerals left me thinking about how these people made others feel: their selflessness, the brilliant families they built, their kindness and their zest for life and fun was celebrated, not their material success or awards.

The changes I've made after these losses:

- The reminder that we never know when our time is going to be up has spurred me into making sure I spend time with the people I really love and value and let them know how much I appreciate them
- Practising gratitude helps us feel more connected and has been shown to be positive for our mental health, all of which should help with that acceptance of mortality Jaques was sure we needed to live a better later life
- On a practical level, I'm trying to make sure my estate is tidy. I know that you are not going anywhere for a long time but no matter how little materially you think you are going to leave, without a will and without making your spouse or a designated other the executor of the estate, you will be leaving someone some mess to sort

out. There are brilliant online will services now, which are cheaper than using a solicitor.

- Depending on how much of a control freak you are, if you have definite ideas about what your funeral and wake should look and feel like, then write those thoughts down. As I say, I know you aren't going anywhere for a long time, but it will save your partner and family a lot of heartache debating what they think you'd like, and I certainly don't want my coffin being carried in to Whitney's 'I Will Always Love You'. I'd be livid.

GOOD GRIEF

It was an honour to welcome psychotherapist Julia Samuel onto the podcast. She's channelled over thirty years of her clinical experience of grief counselling and working with the bereaved into three books on grief and loss, *Grief Works*, *This Too Shall Pass* and *Every Family Has a Story*, and I thought there could be no one better to discuss the changes, fears, losses and healing processes so many of us are faced with in the midlife. She became an expert in this area because of her own experiences with loss.

'All therapists are influenced and do this job from their own experiences. I was brought up in a family where both of my parents were very significantly bereaved way before I was born,' she told me. 'My mum was an orphan; her mother, father, sister and brother had all died tragically and unexpectedly by the time she was twenty-five. And my dad's father and brother had also died unexpectedly, so I was brought up in a house that had lots of great things, but there was this unvoiced grief . . . these black-and-white photographs of very significant grandparents and my aunts and uncles, who were never talked about because my parents were the generation [who thought] what you don't talk about isn't going to hurt you, and I think that made me very curious to know what was going on below the waterline, more interested than what people were saying because we actually never talked about what really mattered. We only talked about what didn't matter. I think being a twin as well, I was always seeking connection. Those two things combined unconsciously. So, when I went on to train as a therapist when I was just thirty, I didn't realise that was the influence, but it didn't take long for me to work that out.'

Many people in midlife are experiencing loss, whether it's parents or friends, but as a society we are clueless about dealing with our grief. We're never taught about grief, and it's one of those emotions that remains taboo, isn't it?

'It really is taboo and I think it scares us. And I think what's interesting about the midlife is not only are our parents maybe given a diagnosis, and grief starts at the point of diagnosis – the minute someone is life threatened, you kind of feel that *Jaws* music of fear that someone I love is going to die – but also midlife, we know there's less ahead than behind, so we feel our mortality more. One of the great fears around grief and death is, If I look at it, is there a kind of magical thinking I'm going to make it happen? If you crack on and pretend everything's okay, then maybe it's not going to catch me.'

Research shows that we have to face our fears, and not be scared to feel the pain of loss, correct?

'Pain is the agent of change. Pain is the thing that forces us to adjust to this new reality that our parent, friend or sibling has died, or is dying. Grief is naturally adaptable. It's meant to adjust our thinking and reality. To face this new reality that this person is no longer physically present. When we block that we block our capacity to feel alive. So, we feel less, and we block our capacity to feel joy. Give yourself space to feel the pain, grieve and emote. Be sad and oscillate to being restorative, to being okay, to getting on to having life in your life, to connecting to others, and giving yourself permission to feel joy. One of the most complicated aspects of grief is guilt. Am I allowed to feel joy? And if we can recognise that guilt is an emotion that we put on ourselves, that doesn't normally come from anybody else. The single biggest predictor of outcomes for people who are grieving is the love and connection of others. When our love for someone who has died is so painful, it is only the love of others that helps us survive.'

Julia's advice on how best to support a loved one dealing with grief

- The most important step is to support them and not try to push them out of it. One of the things to know is that grief tends to take longer than anyone wants. Societally, we give somebody three months or six months or a year and the level of the loss is equal to the level of the emotional investment and the significance of the relationship. So, if this was a death of someone who was really important, that's going to be a long road. So, patience is one of the first things.
- Ask what they need. What do they want? What are they having difficulty with? The biggest thing you can do is listen. You can't fix this. You can't bring the person back. You can't take the pain away. But by offering your love, your connection, your willingness to listen and hear them – and they may well repeat themselves over and over and over – but that will be healing.
- Get outside. I suggest that walking and talking, getting outside, winter or summer, and walking side by side – and maybe with your kids as well, because it is good to model for them that we can be sad, that we grieve, that this is how we manage it. By moving together in

rhythm, you are not eyeballing each other. By the end of
the walk, everybody does feel lighter, and then go and
have a pizza or go home and have a nice lunch.

- There're many different kinds of grief. We don't get over
stuff. We learn to live with it. We learn to accommodate
it and build our life around it. But it's those moments
of love and connection where you really feel seen,
where you really feel you've helped someone that build
the bonds of love in families. I think one of the most
important things to recognise in a family system is
to allow everybody in the family to grieve in their
own particular unique way. The teenage son with his
brother dying may want to just play a lot of football,
be with his mates, kind of be a teenager. The mum
most likely is going to be crying all of the time, and the
dad may be quiet and not be so obviously distressed.
And to recognise that all of those ways of grieving are
completely normal and to allow each of them to express
their grief for themselves. But what helps is finding ways
of coming together to express what they feel. And that
might be something like if you have a box in the sitting
room or in the hall where you have a notepad and pen
and people would write about the son that died and put
a little message in the box and then every month or few
months, or whatever you decide, you sit around together
and you read the messages. Use that as a touchstone to
remember the son that's died and find ways of talking
about it because it's hard.

- Often if you ask somebody how they feel, they shut
down. But if you have a kind of mechanism that allows
you to talk about the person, that is what you want
because you need to both face the reality of the loss and
remember that the love for that person never dies.

- Having touchstones to the memory of (the deceased) and

developing rituals within the family that represent and connect to them are really important. I worked with a family this week whose son died and it's his birthday this weekend, and they're doing two things. They're going to a music event, which is a happy thing as the whole family. Then they're going home and they've got a cake and they're going to have tea and celebrate his birthday. Doing both those things as a family is very collective and collaborative, and everyone can feel their own things. What often splits families is (the idea) there's a right way or wrong way of grieving, but everyone is suffering and they don't know how to communicate or connect with each other, and so they splinter.

- Multiple losses have a compounding effect. One of the ways (to cope) is to boundary time to think about each (loss) individually, otherwise it's overwhelming for your brain to have all of those losses at once. The other thing I would look at is getting proper psychological support because you probably can't manage on your own and it would be helpful for you to get support from a therapist.

- It is never too late to grieve. Research shows that 15 per cent of all psychological disorders come from unresolved grief. So the mindset of 'If I don't feel it, if I don't feel the pain now, I'm going to be okay' is the opposite of the truth. If I allow myself to grieve and feel the pain, paradoxically, that is how I heal and how actually I may even have growth and I'll thrive because we are wired to change. We are wired to accommodate and live with enormous losses and difficulties. But in order to do that, we have to find ways of supporting ourselves to metabolise it and give ourselves opportunities to feel it. And then we can really live and be happy in love again despite these enormous difficulties that all of us at some time in our life will face.

The Midpointer View

Television presenter Richard Bacon had a near-death experience when he was forty-two. 'I was flying home from America and I got a double lung infection – so pneumonia is one lung, double pneumonia is when it hits both lungs and that's when it's very dangerous. I went to Lewisham Hospital, and when you go to hospital and say, "I'm short of breath," they take it very seriously. They rushed me through, did a load of checks, looked at an X-ray and gave me a four-minute warning and said, "It's overtaking your lungs and you're going to die if we don't put you into a coma." I made some quick phone calls to relatives and was asleep.'

He survived, and now lives in Los Angeles with his lovely family, but how has this affected his fear of dying? 'I think it made me more impatient. It's made me think about death a lot. It's quite hard not think about death when you're that close to it. The consultant afterwards said they had expected me to die. I turned blue. They got the crash equipment out, my blood oxygen went below 60 and you're meant to die below 60. And so, I was within seconds of dying and then somehow didn't. I was forty-two when that happened and death still felt distant and abstract and not something to really think about and now, I think about it all the time and maybe that has dovetailed with this sense of urgency of trying to get things done. And so much has happened since then. And I think it is to do with me kind of wanting to sprint at things. I was already impatient, but there's definitely just a sense of wanting to get things done and a realisation that I'm definitely going to die.'

HOW TO TALK TO CHILDREN ABOUT THEIR GRANDPARENTS DYING

Of course, in midlife, most of us are not only worrying about her own ability to cope with pain and grief, but our children's too, as grandparents die, or their friends' parents or grandparents. 'I think one of the natural responses with children and death is that we want to protect them,' explains Julia. 'We don't want them to suffer. We don't want them to be scared; we don't want them to worry. What all the research shows, as well as all the young people I've spoken to, is that in reality, children need the same truth as all of the adults around them, but they need an age-appropriate language. So, if your child asks you, or if you're going to be talking about this kind of thing, you need to use the word dead and dying, like, "Grandpa has died. That means his body doesn't work any more, his heart isn't beating, he's dead." Don't use "gone to heaven", "gone to a better place", "passed away", "lost" – because all of those words, children lose things every day and children live in kind of magical thinking, so they'll think, Oh, well, I can go to heaven. It's the room next door, it's the hamburger joint down the street. I can find my granddad there."

'The basic question I ask all families when someone is dying or has died is: What are your worries? And children are really honest. It could be, "I'm worried, Mum, you're not going to take me to school because you're still crying about Grandpa" or, "Mum, are you going to die?" because they recognise that we're mortal ... And the answer [to your children's question] would be, "I am going to die. It's very unlikely I'm going to die until I'm as old as your grandparents." And that is the truth. You can't promise you're not going to die.'

The Midpointer View

He's known for his strong opinions and being a bit of a loudmouth, but when Piers Morgan came on the podcast, and talked loss and grief, and how a positive attitude can lessen the gloom, we all learnt a few things. 'My first wife was a nurse ward sister, and she really believed in the power of positive thought; that she saw it every day on the wards, that patients could sometimes live or die depending on how positive they were. Not always, obviously, sometimes you're given a terrible situation. It doesn't matter how positive you are, you're going to die. But she saw it every day with people that the power of positive thought can do something to a body that can get you out of a bad situation. Life's tough. It's hard. It's going to throw you difficult stuff, and it's not about how hard you can hit, it's about how hard you can be hit repeatedly and keep moving forward. You get hit, get up and keep marching forward.'

WHEN DIVORCE FEELS LIKE DEATH

I asked Julia about the loss one can feel after a divorce, which often pushes us into a state of grief, and how we can move on when the person is still alive? She describes divorce as living loss. 'I think it's underestimated by people close to you, and society, just how big a loss it is, and that it can feel like a shattering of the dream that you wanted, and a dream that Disney has built for us, a dream that has sold books.'

How can we start to come to terms with it?

'First of all, legitimise and acknowledge how big a loss it is. You will really feel it viscerally, like grief. Divorce is extremely painful because we grieve the future we had every right to expect. Also, with a divorce, it is so complicated. What's yours? What's theirs? What did we do together? All the what ifs? Like, why didn't I or why didn't they? And the confidence that it can really shatter or damage. Will I dare love again? Can I trust again? Am I going to be alone for ever? And then all the ways that you go out in the world – your child's sports day, going to a friend's party – where you are walking in a lane where you used to [walk] as a couple. One of the things for women in particular is you are treated with less respect as a single woman in midlife divorce than you are as a couple. When you go and stay with people, you are given the child's bedroom with the Batman wallpaper, rather than the double that you are given as a couple. I think there's a whole un-conscious societal degrading that divorced women in particular have. And I don't think it's true of divorced men. I think divorced men are seen as catches. When men are widowed, one of the things that people talk about is that men replace and women mourn. And I think in divorce what happens very commonly, men find a new partner very quickly or date very quickly, and women have less people available to them because they have more age difficulties and they take it much harder to find a new partner. It brings up a whole lot of fear. It is a big grief.'

How can we help ourselves feel better after the end of a marriage or a break-up?

'Get exercise, make or maintain lots of connection, eat and sleep well. Put fun front and centre in your new life: whether that's dancing in the kitchen, going for a picnic in the park in the summer or going to a movie, doing things that are simple, not hard to arrange, that give you some joy in your life, but give yourself opportunities to grieve, write it down, talk to friends, maybe see a therapist because it's a painful process and it takes longer than you want. To get through the loss of a relationship or friendship, you need the support of other friends to help to talk it through and to rebuild your confidence in yourself as a friend, as well as let yourself feel sad.'

MIDPOINT ACTION POINTS

- 'Grief works better out loud,' said Doug Manning, a writer, minister and counsellor who wrote about grief and elder care for decades. What is he saying? I think he wants to remind people suffering loss that they are not alone, and they don't need to hide their pain. If you want to, you should talk, share, reminisce, and listen to other people's stories of love and loss.
- Try not to hide or hibernate from the pain you're feeling. Grieving is confronting and awful and hard ... but as a process, it needs to be done eventually. You can't hide from the devastation of losing a loved one or the end of a marriage; you're just pushing your trauma into dark, secret places, or kicking it down the road to wait for you in the future.
- If you're struggling with any kind of loss, do seek help. From your GP, a grief counsellor, your religious guide or friends who have been through similar with wise heads on their shoulders. Don't struggle alone.

16 WORK AND MONEY

... if you work hard enough and assert yourself, and use your mind and imagination, you can shape the world to your desires.

MALCOLM GLADWELL

Work and money appear to be intrinsically linked when you first start your career or accept your first job offer. Very few of us had the luxury at the age of eighteen or twenty-one of choosing a lower-paid job because it afforded us a better lifestyle, or more satisfaction, although today's millennials are certainly more likely to think about how their work life fits in with their mental well-being and free time – and good for them for moving the dial. Us midlifers were part of a generation that almost expected to be exhausted by work. We wanted to get promoted as fast as we could and make money on the way because we wanted to (expected to!) get on the housing ladder by the time we hit our mid to late twenties. Although we hoped to enjoy our work it wasn't a foregone conclusion that we would get job satisfaction. I feel very lucky to have enjoyed a career that has brought me joy, brilliant friendships and some financial security, although I didn't start a pension early enough and instead, Kenny and I relied on flipping property to move up the ladder and build a financial nest egg. We've fallen into that group of people who assume one day they will downsize to release equity but secretly hope they can somehow cobble enough together in their pension to not have to do that.

I don't yet see a time when I will ever completely stop working, which is a common theme among my peer group; very few talk of retiring in the same way our grandparents did. The current age for a state pension is sixty-six years old, and that seems far too young in my mind to be slowing down. That's not to say that the pension age should be raised. I may change my mind, but right now I can't imagine what I would do all day. I like the idea of doing half as much paid work as I do now by the age of sixty-six, but I don't want to be fully put out to grass, which is even more reason to be adhering to the advice of the experts when it comes to diet and lifestyle. Many of my friends have already carved out portfolio careers, consultancy work or started lifestyle businesses which they also seem to combine with more volunteering work, such as being school governors or charity trustees.

I have a great role model in my mum, who at seventy-three years old is still running her property business and thrives on the daily interactions she has with clients and tradespeople. Her job really does keep her young in spirit and she has enormous energy. The relationships we have through work, whether they become friendships or stay purely professional, will go some way to keeping us connected with the world and challenge us mentally. It is not the job per se but the interactions we have which are important, which is why even if you don't work for money any more, it is important to have commitments. You might have to take on a full-time caring role for elderly relatives or grandchildren; you might be doing pro bono work for a charity or organisation you admire – all of these give us connectivity and purpose.

In the 'Blue Zones' (the five regions of the world associated with extraordinary longevity), having a purpose is a common trait and is associated with reduced risk of death through increased psychological well-being. That purpose does not have to be a high-profile career or demanding job but something which forces you into action every day, gives you a routine, gives you a reason to get up, get dressed and get out.

The Midpointer View

Penny Lancaster found a new sense of purpose in midlife thanks to a new career with the police. 'In a position like I am, you always feel like you need to give back and with all the charities and campaigning I do, I never quite felt that it's enough. Now, there's a sense of achievement, there's a sense you've made a difference. And that's what I needed. It felt like it was a natural calling. As scary as it is, chasing down criminals who were threatening to stab you with their hypodermic needle, I've always been one that takes up a challenge and kind of runs towards a danger. We never know until we're put in a life-threatening situation or a scary scenario, whether we're going to be fight, flight or freeze, but I've definitely discovered I'm a fighter. I run to save people, run to take someone down. When you sign up for the police, there's a huge mountain of vetting processes you have to go through and boxes you have to tick and training you have to do. But nowhere does it say you can't be a police officer if you are a rock star's wife. I'm not doing it for the money. I'm volunteering my time just as I would do in any other form of charity. When people think of the police, they think of them as a force, something to be reckoned with, but really a lot of the time our priority is to preserve life, and to protect life and property. Rod's initial reaction was when I did those two weeks in Peterborough, "I've never seen you so excited. It's like me coming off stage after a concert." That resonated with me; we've all got to find something in our life that's meaningful.'

CHANGE CAN DO YOU GOOD

Switching careers in midlife has become much more common, which I suspect might be something to do with the length of time we are going to be expected to work. If the pensionable age keeps on being shifted by a year or two every decade or so, we are probably looking at being aged around seventy by the time we hit that period, so if you 'have' to work until then (according to the government's laws) then a lot of Midpoints are reckoning that they may as well do something they really enjoy or have always had a burning desire to do.

> ### The Midpointer View
>
> Jane Fallon's midpoint now-or-never mindset pushed her to fulfil her childhood ambitions. 'I've had this weird midlife career change. I think I was forty-six when my first book was published. I always had this underlying burning ambition that I'd had since I was a kid, which was to be a novelist. I think I was forty-five [when] I got braver than I'd ever been in my life and decided that now was the time I was going to take time out of work and write a novel. And before that I'd never even told people that it was what I wanted to do. I thought, I'll give myself a year and I'll try and write a book and see what happens. And it worked. I'm on my thirteenth novel now and I started sixteen years ago.'

HOW TO TAKE THE LEAP

If you really want to test your midlife mental performance, then retraining or changing careers might be the ultimate leap of faith. I spoke to Lucy Kellaway – someone who really changed things up in her career at The Midpoint. Lucy was a writer at the *Financial Times* for thirty-two years until she gave it all up to become a teacher. Her midlife pivot involved retraining and then as she enjoyed her new life so much and saw the benefits to the students of having teachers who'd come from different walks of life, she set up an organisation to encourage others to do the same. 'It's called Now Teach and we have had people as old as seventy-one join us and as young as forty-three,' she laughed when we discussed her career change on the podcast. I asked her to share words of encouragement to those of us who would love to do the same.

'Change is weird,' she admitted immediately. 'I had had this very stable life for decades and decades, and I just started chipping away at it, and I made one change and that sort of unblocked me and opened the way to everything else. My big leap was leaving my job as a journalist to become a secondary school teacher. Lots of people thought I was completely nuts but it made perfect sense in that I'd been at the *Financial Times* for thirty-two years. It's just too long. As our lives get longer and longer, the thought you just do one thing? The *FT* was cushy, but as I got older, I stopped caring about the glamour side of it that appealed to me when I was younger, and I thought, How often can a woman repeat herself, writing the same blinking column?'

So how did she come up with the idea of going back to school – and staying there? 'The teaching thing wasn't a great leap of imagination because my mum was an amazing teacher and my oldest daughter left university and she had become a teacher too. I looked at what she was doing with her life and I thought, Actually, you're a lot more useful than I am. And if you can do it, so can I. So that was how it all started.'

But going from the glam life of journalism to a classroom full of fifteen-year-old kids? It sounds hard. 'That is the bit that I was hoping that I would find magic, and I really do. Kids are kids. These ones have very different backgrounds to mine, but connecting with them within the sort of rigidity of school, it's very easy. As soon as you are in there and you are their blinking maths teacher, you have a channel that has been made for you. And people say, "Oh, isn't it horrible if you live so close to your school, and you meet your kids in Sainsbury's?" No! I love meeting my students in Sainsbury's. Even if some of them aren't being terribly nice to you, it makes you feel more optimistic. I think it's very unlikely that there's something special about me. I think that if you are actually interested in young people and show that you are interested, then it's so easy to connect.'

Lucy's practical tips for changing careers at The Midpoint

Lucy has solid advice on this. 'I'm certainly not going to say, "Hey, look at me, I've changed my life. All of you are slightly dissatisfied, just tear the whole thing down." That would be disastrous advice!'

- It's never too late. I first thought of doing this not in my late fifties but in my late forties, and I thought then, Actually, I'm too old to become a teacher. What is so weird is that ten years later, I no longer felt I was too old. I felt I was just right. Changing your life when you are really very late in the day is easier than doing it earlier because you are leaving less behind, oddly, and the stakes are lower.
- There's less to lose. A lot of people say, 'It's so brave what you're doing', and sometimes confronting a really difficult class feels quite brave in the moment, but

changing my life didn't feel very brave because there was
very, very little jeopardy. I wasn't actually giving up very
much by then.

- Remember your value. I've set up a thing now called
Now Teach to try to encourage other middle-aged
people like me to become teachers. And if you change
career in midlife and it doesn't work well, how bad is
that? Now Teach encourages people who have done
other things with their lives to train as teachers and
share all of that experience in the classroom. We had
forty-five people in our first year; the youngest of
whom was 43, the oldest was 71, and we're growing
every year.

A FUNNY EXAMPLE

We have had some great guests on the podcast who have taken
bold steps in midlife, including the brilliant John Bishop who went
from pharmaceutical salesman to stand-up comedian at forty years
old. Today, he is one of the highest-grossing comedians in the UK.
Being at The Midpoint was key to this change. He told me it was
the start of his midlife when he began to ask himself where he was
going and what he was doing. But he has a reminder for midlifers
who want to start afresh. 'Your dreams have to have some base of
reality. You've got to prove you can do it.' He learnt this the hard
way on the comedy circuit. 'When you think about most careers,
if you are applying for a job, somebody's got to approve you. There
might be an interview of one person or an interview board, but
when you're a comedian, you're getting interviewed by 150 people
in the room and therefore it's a real meritocracy because it's instant
communication. As soon as you stop speaking, people laugh or
they don't laugh, that's the end of it.'

I wanted to know if it was easier for John to become famous in middle-age, rather than when he was younger? 'We've been having some conversations with our kids lately and they were saying how confusing it was for them. They were teenage kids who'd had an ordinary bloke, a dad, and then there's somebody famous living in the house. Not all of it was positive, they said, because people expect them to be a mini version of the person that they've seen on the telly. The first year, I didn't make as much and we were having to borrow money against the house to pay for school fees and everything else ... The same with the second year, and the third year. I thought, God, I've got to at least break even in the third year.' Luckily for us, he did – and he didn't have to go back to pharmaceutical sales.

NEVER STOP LEARNING

Pausing a career to take a professional course, a degree or a Master's is often a way people pivot at The Midpoint. I have a forty-two-year-old friend, who was a banker before having children, who has started a Psychology Master's with a view to practising at the end of it, and I'm so proud of her. Your financial position and the dependants in your family will play a huge factor in whether it is even possible to take time out to study, and it may be a tough family decision if the other person in your relationship becomes the sole breadwinner, so it's not a decision to take lightly. But looking at my friend's scenario: she could be a qualified clinical psychologist in a couple of years' time and then have a good twenty-five years of practice to earn good money. If you are harbouring a dream or wanting to hatch a plan to change your career then seize the moment and get advice and you can make this dream a reality.

The Midpointer View

Ruby Wax has really and truly had a wonderfully diverse and interesting journey through her career, but it's her own journey with mental health – about which she's been incredibly outspoken and honest – which has launched her into a new sphere and given her a whole new audience.

Ruby was around fifty when she stopped being on television. I asked her about one of my fears – the idea of being irrelevant! 'You're not allowed on TV after [fifty], it's too upsetting to people. I'm not one of these people to get on a soapbox, and it's just the way it is. They started offering me things like: would I mind going to an island and eating my young? And that's what happens when you're older and when you're very desperate, you end up on those shows. I had to reinvent really quickly. I didn't want to be one of those old people that goes, "Remember me?" and then has people come over and watch reruns or do a documentary about my gallbladder operations.'

How did she handle the end of her career being thrust upon her? 'I had to reinvent. And if I hadn't done that at that age, I wouldn't have ended up getting my Master's and getting whatever else I got. In a way, women have to reinvent constantly because we just live too long. It was primal, my reaction, because it was taking food out of my kids' mouths because I'm the breadwinner. There was a savagery about it. Now how do I survive? It turned out all right against all odds. It's a miracle that you get a job in television, and it's a miracle that at age 107, I got into Oxford when I was an idiot as a child. When I was twenty-one, I wanted to be relevant and I wanted people to pay attention. So I got on TV and showed off – it made up for all my parents going, "You'll never be anything." On the other hand, you can't live with that motive when you're forty.'

MONEY TALKS

I will always regret two things in life: giving up piano lessons and not starting a pension sooner ... which is the most middle-aged thing I think I have ever said! As a freelancer there always seemed to be something else I needed to spend my money on from a mortgage, to a wedding, to school fees, or even a well-deserved holiday, so the pension contributions were never what they should have been. But a few years ago, Kenny and I decided to get a bit more grown up and realised we needed to be more serious about our pension after a financial adviser told me that *I needed to get on with it* in very stern tones.

Pensions and planning

Now there're two words that can make you yawn, correct? But we need to get to grips with our future finances at The Midpoint and who better to give us the crucial information – and push – to start thinking about it than Claer Barrett, the *Financial Times'* Consumer Editor, host of the *FT's Money Clinic with Claer Barrett* podcast and author of the bestselling *What They Don't Teach You About Money*. I got her on *The Midpoint* to share her wisdom, and to tell me what so many of us fear – if we've left it too late to have a good retirement.

'It's never too late to start contributing more to your pension,' she assured me. Phew. 'I think a lot of people are put off by the word pension. They think pensioner. I'm not quite ready to think of myself as an old person yet, they think; this is a problem I can worry about tomorrow. But women especially are likely to have far smaller pension pots than men, partly because it's part of our pay (and women statistically earn less) or if we had a career break to raise children or care for parents, so we need to think about our pensions.' But where to start?

Claer's top tips on the questions you should be asking and the changes you should be making in midlife

- Be aware of what you have. There's over an estimated fifty billion pounds of pensions that have lost touch with their owners. Often people get to the age of fifty and think, Well, what have I got? Because retirement is kind of a bit of a question mark on the horizon when you have a significant birthday. There are all kinds of ways you can track down lost pensions for free online.
- Speak to your HR department or your company bosses, if you have one, to find out what you could get in the future if you paid in a bit more today. If you sacrifice a small amount more of your salary, the employers often offer match contributions. Maybe if you pay in 5 per cent, they'll pay in 10 per cent, but you could opt to pay in 6 per cent and they would pay in 12 per cent. Getting these little incremental increases over time can compound, your investments will grow and that could put you in a better position.
- We also need to talk about pensions with our partners. I often challenge *FT* readers to find out what their personal gender pension gap is. By which I mean what's your pension or your pensions, what collectively are they worth, and what are your partner's pensions collectively

worth? Because it's bound to be a figure that neither of you really know the answer to. And often people are really shocked by the impact taking a career break to care for others has had. Women's pensions are often quite minuscule. And it may be that you can solve this as a partnership, either by your partner paying more into your pension, setting up a private pension for you going forward, or just making it possible for you to contribute more from your salary so that things can be equalised.

- If you are structured as a sole trader, you don't have as many pension options as you do if you are a limited company. It's well worth speaking to your accountant about this if you are self-employed because as a limited company director, your company can pay a percentage of the profits that you are making tax-free into your pension as a company contribution. Lots of self-employed people don't realise this is possible and need a little bit of financial advice to help make a plan going forward about how to be taxed as efficiently as possible. How could I get the most money out of the government? Put something aside. It's not anything that we are taught in schools or even in business schools, but it really should be because it could make a difference.

- My final point on finances and pensions in the midlife is about divorce. You could be all right with a partner, have owned a house, have paid off the mortgage, but then if you decide to become a silver splitter, as the trend is known because older divorce is on the rise, then you've got to find the money for two separate households and life's going to get a lot more expensive and complicated. Plus, when people get divorced, the pension isn't taken into consideration. But gold-plated company pensions that people (mostly men) in their fifties and sixties have may well be worth more than the value of the family

home. In so many divorces, pensions are not taken
into consideration as part of the split and that's a crime
against women's finances. I think surfacing it and raising
awareness of it has to be the first step.

Money guru Claer's parting piece of advice is to be realistic
about your financial future. 'Retirement has changed,' she reminds
us. 'It's not this hard stop that it used to be. People want to carry
on working part time, or maybe in a consultancy capacity if they're
lucky enough to be able to do that. I think we will see people pivot
their careers as they get older to get into work they could keep
doing for longer. We all need to invest in ourselves to upskill, to
look at what's happening, to think, Would I be better off in my late
career shifting to a different department, thinking strategically:
where could I get those plum kind of jobs? How could I shift into
a more freelance lifestyle as I age? These are all things that need to
be front of mind when you are in your fifties.

FUTURE PERFECT?

You may be reading this chapter thinking that I am an idiot for
being so relaxed about planning for our future or you might be
feeling a kinship and wondering if it is too late to get yourself
something started for your older age. If you are the latter group,
I would suggest you speak to a professional. I know it can be a
little scary if money matters are not your comfy place, but they
will help you work out if making provisions for the future and
investing in pensions is something you can afford to start now.
Seriously: make it a priority. It's never too late to plan ahead, but
the sooner the better.

MIDPOINT ACTION POINTS

- There's a popular saying that if you find a job you love, you will never work a day in your life. However true this may be, it is not realistic for most of us – so look for aspects you love in a job that may still feel like work. Does it encourage you to learn new skills, meet new people, travel? Do you have a laugh with your colleagues, meet people you'd never normally get to meet, feel you've achieved something at the end of the day? Take the positives out of work, and fill in the missing parts with hobbies and pastimes.

- Do your research. It can be a difficult thing to discuss with your partner – or your bank manager – but you need to talk about money. Think about working with a financial adviser to work out what you've got . . . and what you'll need in the future. Knowledge is power.

- Money makes the world go around, but it doesn't bring limitless happiness with it. Remember that: don't only think about your bank balance when you're making choices for yourself and your loved ones.

EPILOGUE: LIFE IS BEAUTIFUL

Well, it's nothing very special. Uh, try and be nice to
people, avoid eating fat, read a good book every now and
then, get some walking in, and try and live together in
peace and harmony with people of all creeds and nations.

MONTY PYTHON'S THE MEANING OF LIFE

Since I turned fifty my life has been full of unexpected moments of gratitude. It wasn't that I felt ungrateful before but maybe I was more expectant, in my teens, twenties and thirties, that life would work out how I hoped it would and everything would fall into place. It's only now, when I step back and look at what I have built and created in my life so far, I realise it's a minor miracle I got here in one piece, with people I love and care about. Yes, that is what reliving my journey to The Midpoint – and through it – on the previous pages of this book has made me feel: grateful. I see the midlife as a time we can lean in and explore the things that give us emotional satisfaction a bit more purposefully, and I hope this book has helped you do that, too. When we are rushing through the building careers and family decades, we might not have the time to stop to pay full attention to friendships, or our health, or our marriage. Now is the time we should reclaim a bit of care and attention for ourselves. We must.

I started making *The Midpoint* podcast because I was sparked by a revelation one day when I walked past a mirror. Inside, I still felt twenty-eight, but my reflection stopped me in my tracks. I was shocked to see, staring back at me, a middle-aged woman. And what do I do with that? What did that mean for me, my body, my brain, my career? Society is not known for being kind to people over the age of forty-five, especially women.

One of my podcast guests, Caitlin Moran, talked to me about her own realisation of her middle-age-dom, and how she embraced it. 'I started looking in history,' she told me. 'The three phases in a woman's life are the maid or virgin, then the mother, and then you go to crone, witch, hag, then you're dead. So, I researched the lives of hags, crones and witches, and decided I wanted a hag life. Hags lived in houses in the forest. They were intolerant of stupid people. They stomped around in their cloaks with their staffs, while they tended their garden, grew their herbs, made their potions, and did wild rituals in the woods, jumping into lakes and cackling with their fellow crones, witches and hags – and people left them alone and respected them.'

When it's explained like that, being at The Midpoint sounds wonderfully empowering, doesn't it? It should. Because it can be. My experts and guests have taught me that time and time again.

Do one last thing for me. Fast forward to your deathbed. Imagine you're taking your last breaths. What will you wish you spent more *or* less time doing? Who will you wish you spent more *or* less time with? You may regret not looking after your health, prioritising work, staring at your phone too much. You probably won't regret gawping at a sunset, telling your people how much you love them, travelling to places that made your heart soar. Start living with these realisations today, at The Midpoint. You may feel like middle age is too late, but it isn't. You could still have decades of healthy, happy years in front of you. Don't sell yourself short.

Take the teachings you've learnt from everything you've been through so far, and implement them into your current midlife. Learn to accept what you love, and what you don't. Try new things, no matter how silly they sound or out of character they feel. You are not too old to make changes. Regular sunrise swims or setting yourself a 100-book per year challenge could bring meaning to your midpoint life in simple, unexpected ways. Value authenticity and stop wasting time with people or pastimes that don't bring genuine joy. When you truly know yourself, you can grow yourself ... and your midpoint (and beyond) will be marvellous. Good luck.

ACKNOWLEDGEMENTS

The first thank you has to go to all the wonderful contributors to *The Midpoint* podcast. As I write we have produced over 100 episodes, with such a wide variety of guests, from Olympic gold medal winners to stand-up comedians and Hollywood actresses to famous vicars – and in all that time I have been thrilled at how open and honest my guests have been. These interviews sparked the idea for this book, and I am so grateful for the time my contributors gave up and for their generosity in letting me share their musings.

Thank you also to the experts from the podcast, who have given us such a brilliant insight into what we need to do to help our minds, bodies, relationships and finances stay healthy as we head into the next period of life. We all face different challenges and come at this from different perspectives and experiences, but I can honestly say that there hasn't been one conversation that hasn't taught me something and left me better informed, and as we know carrying on learning is one of the golden rules of ageing successfully.

Thank you so much to Sarah Ivens for helping me to make sense of all of this information and for getting the book into great shape. Thank you also to Gina Luck at Piatkus for your brilliant support.

FURTHER RESEARCH

BOOKS I'VE LOVED AND LEARNT FROM . . .

Amati, Dr Federica, *Every Body Should Know This: The Science of Eating for a Lifetime of Health*

Arif, Dr Nighat, *The Knowledge: Your Guide to Female Health – From Menstruation to the Menopause*

Attia, Dr Peter, *Outlive: The Science and Art of Longevity*

Barnett, Jennifer and Willett, Alexis, *How Much Brain Do We Really Need?*

Barrett, Claer, *What They Don't Teach You About Money: Seven Habits to Unlock Financial Independence*

Beeny, Sarah, *The Simple Life: How I Found Home*

Bottley, Rev Kate, *Have A Little Faith: Lessons on Love, Death and How Lasagne Always Helps*

Campbell, Pippa, *Eat Right, Lose Weight: Your Individual Blueprint for Long-term Weight Loss and Better Health*

Candy, Lorraine, *Mum, What's Wrong with You?: 101 Things Only Mothers of Teenage Girls Know*

Chiles, Adrian, *The Good Drinker: How I Learned to Love Drinking Less*

Clear, James, *Atomic Habits: An Easy & Proven Way to Build Good Habits & Break Bad Ones*

Daly, Tess, *4 Steps: To a Happier, Healthier You*

Day, Elizabeth, *How to Fail: Everything I've Ever Learned from Things Going Wrong*

Dondos, Dr Vicky, *The Positive Ageing Plan: The Expert Guide to Healthy, Beautiful Skin at Every Age*

Edmonds, Frances, *Repotting Your Life: Reframe Your Thinking. Reset Your Purpose. Rejuvenate Yourself Time and Again*

Falconer, Jenni, *Runner's High: How to Squeeze the Joy from Every Step*

Fox, Jason, *Embrace the Chaos: 52 Tactics to Make Every Day Count*

Frostrup, Mariella, *Cracking the Menopause: While Keeping Yourself Together*

Grange, Dr Pippa, *Fear Less: How to Win at Life Without Losing Yourself*

Gunter, Dr Jen, *The Menopause Manifesto: Own Your Health with Facts and Feminism*

Harper, Dr Shahzadi and Bardwell, Emma, *The Perimenopause Solution: Take Control of Your Hormones Before They Take Control of You*

Hibbert, Noor, *You Only Live Once: Find Your Purpose. Reclaim Your Power. Make Life Count.*

Hirons, Caroline, *Skincare: The Ultimate No-Nonsense Guide*

Jensen, Frances E., MD, *The Teenage Brain: A Neuroscientist's Survival Guide to Raising Adolescents and Young Adults*

Kellaway, Lucy, *Re-Educated: Why It's Never Too Late to Change Your Life*

Kenny, Professor Rose Anne, *Age Proof: The New Science of Living a Longer and Healthier Life*

Khan, Dr Amir, *The Doctor Will See You Now: The Highs and Lows of My Life as an NHS GP*

Knight, Annabelle, *The Matchmaker's Match*

Lambert, Rhiannon, *The Science of Nutrition: Debunk the Diet Myths and Learn How to Eat Well for Health and Happiness*

Leeming, Dr Emily, *Genius Gut: The Life-Changing Science of Eating for Your Second Brain*

Levy, Miranda, *The Insomnia Diaries: How I Learned to Sleep Again*

McCall, Davina with Dr Naomi Potter, *Menopausing: The Positive Roadmap to Your Second Spring*

Minchin, Louise, *Fearless: Adventures with Extraordinary Women*

Moran, Caitlin, *More Than a Woman*

Newson, Dr Louise, *The Definitive Guide to the Perimenopause & Menopause*

Ong, Simon Alexander, *Energize: Make the Most of Every Moment*

Pink, Matt, *Better ME, Better YOU: Sharing My Journey to Help You Live a Better Life*

Ramlakhan, Dr Nerina, *Tired But Wired: How to Overcome Your Sleep Problems – The Essential Sleep Toolkit*

Roberts, Adele, *Personal Best: From Rock Bottom to the Top of the World*

Rowe-Ham, Kate, *Owning Your Menopause: Fitter, Calmer, Stronger in 30 Days*

Ryder, Amanda, *Feel Good for Menopause: Essential Nutrition and Lifestyle Advice to Support a Healthy Body and Mind*

Samuel, Julia, *Grief Works: Stories of Life, Death and Surviving*

Samuel, Julia, *This Too Shall Pass: Stories of Change, Crisis and Hopeful Beginnings*

Samuel, Julia, *Every Family Has a Story*

Schofield, Rachel, *The Career Change Guide: Five Steps to Finding Your Dream Job*

Shulman, Alexandra, *Clothes... And Other Things That Matter*

Spargo-Mabbs, Fiona, *I Wish I'd Known: Young People, Drugs and Decisions: A Guide for Parents and Carers*

Steele, Andrew, *Ageless: The New Science of Getting Older Without Getting Old*

Taylor, Davinia, *It's Not a Die: The No Cravings, No Willpower Way to Get Lean and Happy for Good*

Taylor, Davinia, *Hack Your Hormones: Effortless Weight Loss. Better Focus. Deeper Sleep. More Energy.*

Thaler, Richard H and Sunstein, Cass R, *Nudge: Improving Decisions About Health, Wealth and Happiness*

Thomas, Gareth, *Stronger*

Van Tulleken, Dr Chris, *Ultra Processed People: Why Do We All Eat Stuff That Isn't Food.. .and Why Can't We Stop?*

Wax, Ruby, *A Mindfulness Guide for Survival*

Whyte, Professor Greg, *Achieve the Impossible*

Winkleman, Claudia, *Quite*

Young, Will, *Be Yourself and Happier: The A-Z of Wellbeing*

INSTAGRAM ACCOUNTS THAT EASE MY MIDLIFE MIND AND MAKE ME LAUGH TOO . . .

carolinescircuits

claerb (money expert)

dj_fattony_

dr.fede.amati

dr_idz

emmanevillethisisme

graceghanem

green.edit_

Iceman_hof

Juliasamuelmbe

katerh_fitness

Mamastillgotit_

menopause_doctor

myeasytherapy

pippacampbell_health

postcardsfrommidlife

runna_coach

sineadmckeefry

susannahconstantine

thesecurerelationship

INDEX